THE **BLOOD SUGAR SOLUTION**

10-DAY
DETOX
DIET
COOKBOOK

ALSO BY MARK HYMAN, MD

The Blood Sugar Solution 10-Day Detox Diet

The Blood Sugar Solution Cookbook

The Blood Sugar Solution

The Daniel Plan

The Daniel Plan Cookbook

UltraPrevention

UltraMetabolism

The Five Forces of Wellness (CD)

The UltraMetabolism Cookbook

The UltraThyroid Solution

The UltraSimple Diet

The UltraSimple Challenge (DVD)

The UltraMind Solution

Six Weeks to an UltraMind (CD)

UltraCalm (CD)

THE **BLOOD SUGAR SOLUTION**

10-DAY DETOX DIET COOKBOOK

More than 150 Recipes to Help You Lose Weight and Stay Healthy for Life

Mark Hyman, MD

LITTLE, BROWN AND COMPANY

New York   Boston   London

This book is intended to supplement, not replace, the advice of a trained health professional. If you know or suspect that you have a health problem, you should consult a health professional. The author and publisher specifically disclaim any liability, loss, or risk, personal or otherwise, that is incurred as a consequence, directly or indirectly, of the use and application of any of the contents of this book.

Little, Brown and Company
Hachette Book Group
1290 Avenue of the Americas, New York, NY 10104
littlebrown.com

First Edition: March 2015

Little, Brown and Company is a division of Hachette Book Group, Inc. The Little, Brown name and logo are trademarks of Hachette Book Group, Inc.

The publisher is not responsible for websites (or their content) that are not owned by the publisher.

The Hachette Speakers Bureau provides a wide range of authors for speaking events. To find out more, go to hachettespeakersbureau.com or call (866) 376-6591.

ISBN 978-0-316-33881-3
Library of Congress Control Number: 2014958504

10 9 8 7 6 5 4 3 2

LSC-C

Printed in the United States of America

*For the generations of Americans who never learned to cook
or to care for and nourish their precious human bodies,
this book is for you.*

Contents

Introduction: What Is the 10-Day Detox Diet?   3

PART I

THE BASICS

1. Why Detox?   9
2. Getting Started   16
3. Why Cook?   22
4. Creating a Healing Kitchen   31
5. Tips and Tools   52
6. How to Prepare Simple Meals   58

PART II

THE RECIPES

7. The Basic Plan   63

   Breakfast   64
   Lunch   85
   Dinner   131
   Vegetables and Side Dishes   252
   Snacks   272
   Sauces and Condiments   289
   Spices, Rubs, and Stocks   300

Contents

8. **Healthy Meal Plans**   **305**

   Acknowledgments   309
   Resources   311
   General Index   321
   Recipe Index   329

THE **BLOOD SUGAR SOLUTION**

10-DAY DETOX DIET

COOKBOOK

What Is the 10-Day Detox Diet?

If you're one of the millions of Americans suffering from obesity, diabetes, high blood pressure, or even just plain feeling crummy as a result of the Standard American Diet (SAD), *The Blood Sugar Solution 10-Day Detox Diet* is for you. It provides a step-by-step guide for losing weight and even reversing disease. Follow it for just ten days and your life will never be the same!

The 10-Day Detox Diet outlines a way of eating that will help you reverse the food addiction brought on by the $1-trillion industrial food system—the system that turns sugar, salt, and fat into druglike foods that hook you with every bite. This steady stream of hyperprocessed, highly palatable, intensely addictive foods sabotages your brain chemistry, your waistline, and your health. The way to reclaim your health and your life starts with what I call food rehab. It means a dramatic shift, but it will provide you with the fundamental skills you need to lose weight, change your biochemistry, and kick your addiction forever!

In a recent study, Harvard professor Dr. David Ludwig explains why for the first time. It turns out that it's not overeating that makes you fat; it's being fat that makes you overeat. When you consume refined carbohydrates such as bread, rice, potatoes, pasta, and any form of sugar, you make a certain kind of fat called *visceral adipose tissue* (VAT). This is no ordinary fat. It is super fat. Hungry fat. Dangerous fat. This fat starts an inexorable cascade that leads to obesity. It's like falling down an icy slope where it's almost impossible to stop yourself. We ordinary mortals are no match for this hungry fat.

Here's what happens: VAT cells suck up much of the available fuel in your bloodstream (glucose, fats, ketones). Your body then thinks, "Oh, jeez, I am starving. I better eat more and slow my metabolism, so I don't die." The problem is that anything you eat gets sucked up into those fat cells around your belly, leading to a vicious cycle of hunger, overeating, fat storage, and a slowing down of your metabolism. No wonder we gain weight and can't lose it.

The key trigger for all of this is a hormone that we all need, albeit in moderation: insulin — the fat storage hormone.

If we make too much insulin, it drives the fuel from our blood into our fat cells. Too much insulin also does a lot of other bad things, such as cause heart attacks, high cholesterol, type 2 diabetes, cancer, and dementia.

What causes insulin to spike? Not all calories are created equal: Sugar and refined carbohydrate calories are the culprits. Most Americans eat, on average, about 152 pounds of sugar and 146 pounds of flour a year (combined, that's almost a pound of sugar and flour per person, per day).

The Blood Sugar Solution 10-Day Detox Diet is scientifically designed to stop this vicious cycle quickly. Think of it as your ice axe and crampons to halt your descent down the slippery slope of obesity and chronic disease. It will quickly block the hormones and brain chemicals that make you hungry and crave sugar and carbs. And instead of storing fat and being burdened with a slow metabolism, you will burn fat and speed up your metabolism.

Once you enjoy all of the healing benefits of the 10-Day Detox Diet, my guess is that you'll want to incorporate many of the elements into your life. That's why I've written this cookbook: to review the principles of the program and help support you with information and recipes so you can continue on your path to good health. After all, food is medicine, and I believe you'll find that it's even more powerful than anything you will find in a pill bottle.

The recipes in this book follow the principles of the 10-Day Detox

Diet. I have also included recipes for you to enjoy when the ten days are over—during what I call the "transition phase." After all, better health doesn't start and end in ten days. It's a lifelong journey. I've set out to make that journey both doable and delicious.

Eat Well for Less

Living a healthy life shouldn't be as costly or difficult as it is. I want to share a new resource with you — something that makes eating healthy just as easy and affordable as eating conventional food. Thrive Market is a new online marketplace that sells over 3,000 natural products and healthy foods at wholesale prices by using a membership-club model. By paying less than $5 a month ($59.95 annually), Thrive Market members can find high-quality, natural foods your body needs at prices everyone can afford (25 to 50 percent below retail prices, every day). Stocking a healthy kitchen has truly never been easier.

Your healthy choices don't just benefit you; they help create a society where good health is the norm. Too many families live in food deserts where they simply can't find healthy food. Thrive Market is doing something to help that, too. When you sign up for a new Thrive Market membership, they will donate a free membership to a family in need. This company is democratizing access to healthy food and products, one membership at a time.

Thrive Market wants more people like you to join the movement toward a healthier future — and that's why they're offering everyone reading this book a free two-month membership.

To get your complementary two-month membership, please visit thrv.me/10day.

PART I

THE BASICS

Many of you who have picked up this cookbook may have already read *The Blood Sugar Solution 10-Day Detox Diet* and have experienced the profound effects of resetting your metabolism using food as medicine. I hope you now are addicted not to sugar but to feeling good and you are looking for additional recipes, meal ideas, and encouragement to help you stay on track and maintain the amazing way you feel now.

1

Why Detox?

For those of you who struggle with weight, who are skinny on the outside but fat on the inside, or who have FLC (feel like crap) syndrome, food addiction is often at the root. Addiction to sugar, flour, and processed foods hijacks your life and leads to metabolic chaos—increasing cravings and hunger, slowing metabolism, and packing on belly fat. Although the idea of a detox may sound extreme, I strongly believe that it is the only way to balance your hormones and blood sugar, reduce insulin spikes, cool off inflammation, improve digestion, and boost your metabolism. Think of it as a delicious, energy-boosting, scientific method for detoxing from foods high in sugars and refined carbohydrates and processed food.

We tracked more than 600 people who tried the 10-Day Detox Diet program and found that they experienced dramatic results. On average they lost 8 pounds and 3.4 percent of their body weight, 2 inches off their waist, and 1 inch off their hips. Some people lost up to 10 inches around their waist, and up to 11 inches around their hips. The average drop in fasting blood sugar was 18 points. The average blood pressure fell 10 points. Even better, they had more energy, reported better sleep, and experienced improvements in their mood. They had a 62 percent reduction in symptoms from all diseases. There is no drug on the planet that can do that. One seventy-year-old man told me he lost 45 pounds, got off 52 units of insulin, and completely reversed his diabetes. Another told me his rheumatoid arthritis went away in ten days, and yet another reported that her daily migraines had vanished. These results came not from pill bottles but from food.

In the following pages, I feature three quizzes that will help you identify if you are addicted to food in any way, or if your relationship to food is interfering with the quality of your life, or if food is doing anything other than helping you thrive and feel amazing. If so, then you need this detox. If you have *diabesity*—the continuum of metabolic damage ranging from a little belly fat to pre-diabetes to type 2 diabetes, or if you just don't feel well, then the 10-Day Detox Diet can profoundly improve your health and the quality of your life. And because I encourage you to keep track of your progress during the detox, you will see the results right away.

ARE YOU A FOOD ADDICT?

I'm fed up with the food giants and even many health professionals who perpetuate the myth that a calorie is a calorie—that the 500 calories you wolf down in a Big Mac have the same impact on your body as 500 calories of broccoli. Not all calories are equal. Calories from sugar and refined carbs spike blood sugar, trigger insulin, and lead to a cascade of hormonal and brain chemistry changes that promote fat storage, hunger, and a slow metabolism. Science also supports the notion that your Big Mac, Double Gulp, and other hyperprocessed fat, sugar, and salt bombs are addictive.

While at Yale's Rudd Center for Food Policy and Obesity, my friend and colleague Kelly Brownell, PhD, created a scientifically validated food questionnaire to help you determine whether you are a food addict. I've adapted the quiz below.

QUIZ: Are You Addicted to Food?

Ask yourself how often you experience any of these feelings and behaviors (hint: the more often you experience them, the more addicted you are):

- You consume certain foods even if you are not hungry, because of cravings.

- You worry about cutting down on certain foods.
- You feel sluggish or fatigued from overeating.
- You have spent time dealing with negative feelings from overeating certain foods, instead of spending time in important activities with family, friends, work, or recreation.
- You have had withdrawal symptoms such as agitation and anxiety when you've cut down on certain foods (do not include caffeinated drinks such as coffee, tea, or energy drinks).
- Your behavior with respect to food and eating causes you significant distress.
- Issues related to food and eating decrease your availability to function effectively (daily routine, job/school, social or family activities, health difficulties).
- You need more and more of the foods you crave to experience any pleasure or to reduce negative emotions.

If you see yourself in these clues, don't worry—you're far from alone. Millions of people in every corner of the world have fallen into the food addiction trap. The 10-Day Detox Diet helps you discover once and for all the path that leads you out of biochemical imprisonment and into food freedom. This cookbook helps support you on your journey.

DO YOU HAVE DIABESITY?

As if food addiction isn't destructive enough on its own, the industrial foods that have this druglike effect can also lead to diabesity. Type 2 diabetes now affects one in two American adults (and one in four kids).

In the following quiz, you'll discover whether you're suffering from the symptoms of pre-diabetes or type 2 diabetes—inflammation, high triglycerides, unhealthy cholesterol levels, high blood pressure, and high blood sugar. If you answer "yes" to even one of the following questions, you may already have diabesity or are headed in that direction.

QUIZ: Do I Have Diabesity?

1. Do you have a family history of diabetes, heart disease, or obesity?
2. Are you of nonwhite ancestry (African, Asian, Native American, Pacific Islander, Hispanic, Indian, Middle Eastern)?
3. Are you overweight (body mass index, or BMI, over 25)? Go to www.10daydetox.com/tools to calculate your BMI based on your weight and height.
4. Do you have extra belly fat? Is your waist circumference greater than 35 inches for women or greater than 40 inches for men?
5. Do you crave sugar and refined carbohydrates?
6. Do you have trouble losing weight on a low-fat diet?
7. Has your doctor told you that your blood sugar is a little high (greater than 100 mg/dL) or have you actually been diagnosed with insulin resistance, pre-diabetes, or type 2 diabetes?
8. Do you have high levels of triglycerides (over 100 mg/dL) or low levels of HDL ("good") cholesterol (under 50 mg/dL)?
9. Do you have heart disease?
10. Do you have high blood pressure?
11. Are you inactive (less than 30 minutes of exercise 4 times a week)?
12. Do you suffer from infertility, low sex drive, or sexual dysfunction?
13. For women: Have you had gestational diabetes or polycystic ovarian syndrome (PCOS)?

ARE YOU SICK?

You'll also want to find out just how sick you are by taking the Toxicity Quiz (adapted from the Immuno Symptom Checklist created in 1989 by Immuno Laboratories). Most of us walk around tolerating chronic symptoms (not just weight issues) that are connected to what we eat, including digestive issues, headaches, joint pain, fatigue, depression, autoimmune diseases, and more. Most of us just don't connect the dots. If we eat crap, we will feel like crap. This quiz will give you a baseline for your existing symptoms, which are indications of being toxic and inflamed. Score it now and again after you've completed the program, and you will experience for yourself, after just ten days, a dramatic difference in the way you look and feel.

For the "before" part of the questionnaire, rate each of the following symptoms based upon your health profile for the past 30 days.

Point Scale

0 = Never or almost never have the symptom
1 = Occasionally have it, effect is not severe
2 = Occasionally have, effect is severe
3 = Frequently have it, effect is not severe
4 = Frequently have it, effect is severe

Digestive Tract

_____ Nausea or vomiting
_____ Diarrhea
_____ Constipation
_____ Bloated feeling
_____ Belching or passing gas
_____ Heartburn
_____ Intestinal/stomach pain
Total before _____
Total after _____

Ears

_____ Itchy ears
_____ Earaches or ear infections
_____ Drainage from ear
_____ Ringing or hearing loss
Total before _____
Total after _____

Emotions

_____ Mood swings
_____ Anxiety, fear, or nervousness
_____ Anger, irritability, or aggressiveness
_____ Depression
Total before _____
Total after _____

Energy/Activity

_____ Fatigue or sluggishness
_____ Apathy or lethargy
_____ Hyperactivity
_____ Restlessness
Total before _____
Total after _____

Eyes

_____ Watery or itchy eyes
_____ Swollen, reddened, or sticky eyelids
_____ Bags or dark circles under eyes
_____ Blurred or tunnel vision (does not include near- or farsightedness)
Total before _____
Total after _____

Head

_____Headaches

_____Faintness

_____Dizziness

_____Insomnia

Total before _____

Total after _____

Heart

_____Irregular or skipped
heartbeat

_____Rapid or pounding
heartbeat

_____Chest pain

Total before _____

Total after _____

Joints/Muscles

_____Pain or aches in joints

_____Arthritis

_____Stiffness or limitation of
movement

_____Pain or aches in muscles

_____Feeling of weakness or
tiredness

Total before _____

Total after _____

Lungs

_____Chest congestion

_____Asthma or bronchitis

_____Shortness of breath

_____Difficulty breathing

Total before _____

Total after _____

Mind

_____Poor memory

_____Confusion or poor
comprehension

_____Poor concentration

_____Poor physical coordination

_____Indecisiveness

_____Stuttering or stammering

_____Slurred speech

_____Learning disabilities

Total before _____

Total after _____

Mouth/Throat

_____Chronic coughing

_____Gagging or frequent need
to clear throat

_____Sore throat, hoarseness, or
loss of voice

_____Swollen or discolored
tongue, gums, or lips

_____Canker sores

Total before _____

Total after _____

Nose

_____Stuffy nose

_____Sinus problems

_____Hay fever

_____Excessive mucus formation

_____Sneezing attacks

Total before _____

Total after _____

Skin

_____ Acne

_____ Hives, rashes, or dry skin

_____ Hair loss

_____ Flushing or hot flashes

_____ Excessive sweating

Total before _____

Total after _____

Weight

_____ Binge eating/drinking

_____ Craving certain foods

_____ Excessive weight

_____ Compulsive eating

_____ Water retention

_____ Underweight

Total before _____

Total after _____

Other

_____ Frequent illness

_____ Frequent or urgent urination

_____ Genital itch or discharge

Total before _____

Total after _____

Grand Total Before _____

Grand Total After _____

Key to Questionnaire

Optimal health: less than 10

Mild toxicity: 10–50

Moderate toxicity: 50–100

Severe toxicity: over 100

2

Getting Started

The antidote to your weight and health problems doesn't lie in the pharmacy—it lies, as I have always said, in the "farmacy." The foods in your farmers' market and supermarket hold the cure, and the 10-Day Detox Diet is the way to break the cycle and reset, reboot, and restore your body to good health. This companion cookbook will support you in your mission. It will help you reconnect with your kitchen and prepare real, whole, delicious meals for yourself and those you love.

There are three phases of the 10-Day Detox Diet, all keys to your life-long success. This cookbook will enhance your experience by providing you with more than 150 mouthwatering recipes to give your metabolism a boost. Let's look at the three phases:

Phase 1, the Prep Phase: Here you'll clean out your fridge and pantry in order to set yourself up for success. Spend about two days prior to beginning your detox setting up both mentally and physically. We'll get to specific foods and ingredients in Chapter 4.

Phase 2, the 10-Day Detox: This is the actual "meat" of the program—the ten days that you'll spend resetting your biochemistry and jumpstarting the healing process.

Phase 3, the Transition Phase: Now you'll learn strategies for long-term health so you can continue to feel great after the first ten days.

I've organized the meals in this cookbook to help your body progress according to the same guidelines I outlined in *The Blood Sugar Solution 10-Day Detox Diet*. My dream is for you to follow the comprehensive program in that book and give your body the best chance to reset itself to health. However, if you've picked up this cookbook and want to start with food as your medicine, then you will still experience profound changes in your weight, health, and well-being in just ten days.

WHY 10 DAYS?

Ten days is not a magic number or a gimmicky weight-loss scheme. Most people don't realize that they are only a few days away from health and happiness. When you rapidly shift the way you eat, you can shift your hormones, brain chemistry, and biology very quickly. You can normalize your blood sugar, restore your liver and pancreas to a healthier state, and even improve your metabolism. Your body is capable of amazing things if you give it a chance. Just try it for ten days. You are capable of doing anything for that amount of time. And in exchange for a radical change in your lifestyle, I'm offering you a radical promise: that you will emerge within the first week feeling lighter, happier, more energetic, and more alive. You'll also be released from the grip of food addiction, and your body will be less toxic than it has been in years. Within this cookbook, you'll find the recipes and tools you need to free yourself from the cravings and health struggles that plague you.

WHAT TO TRACK

Throughout your ten-day journey and beyond, I encourage you to track your results. Research shows that people who track their results lose twice as much weight and do twice as well. Begin by getting a journal; it could be as simple as a notebook or a spreadsheet on your computer, whatever is convenient and works for you.

Now, what should you track? For starters, you'll want to get a baseline of all measurements. Before you begin, talk with your healthcare provider about the program if you're already on medication for high blood pressure or high blood sugar. If you are, the diet can work so quickly that your blood sugar or blood pressure may drop significantly — one patient had her sugar drop from 220 to normal in three days. So it is important to work with your doctor to adjust your medication and keep close track of these measurements. Using a home glucose monitor and blood pressure cuff can help you keep close tabs on how your body responds to this healing way of eating. Check out www.10daydetox.com/tools for my recommendations for self-tracking and monitoring devices that track weight, exercise, blood pressure, blood sugar, and more.

Here's a list of what to record, how often to recheck, and what you need to get started:

YOUR WEIGHT

Weigh yourself, without clothes, first thing in the morning after going to the bathroom. Track your weight weekly in your journal.

YOUR HEIGHT

Measure yourself in feet and inches. Write it in your journal.

YOUR WAIST SIZE

Measure the widest point around your belly button. Track this measurement weekly in your journal. You can also track your hips at the widest point around your butt.

YOUR BODY MASS INDEX (BMI)

Your BMI is your weight in kilograms divided by your height in meters squared. You can use our online calculator at www.10daydetox.com/tools or use this calculation:

BMI = weight in pounds times 703, then divided by height in inches squared

So let's use me for example: I weigh 185 pounds and am 75 inches tall. The calculation is: $185 \times 703 \div (75 \times 75)$. My BMI is 23.

This gives you a way to track whether you are normal weight, overweight, or obese. Normal BMI is less than 25, overweight is 26 to 29, and obese is over 30. However, you should take into account your waist size as well. If you weigh a lot but are a muscular bodybuilder with a small waist, you could be healthy and still have a high BMI. If you have skinny arms and legs and a skinny butt but a potbelly, you might have a normal BMI but be at risk for diabesity.

Furthermore, certain ethnic groups—such as Asians, Hispanics, Pacific Islanders, Inuits, Indians, and Middle Easterners—have diabesity at much lower BMIs. Track your BMI weekly in your journal.

YOUR BLOOD PRESSURE (optional)

Get a home blood pressure cuff and measure your blood pressure first thing every morning and write it down.

WHAT TESTS SHOULD YOU DO?

Test Your Blood Sugar Yourself

While measuring your blood sugar is optional before, during, and after the 10-Day Detox Diet, I highly recommend it. Many people think they don't have to check their blood sugar unless they are diabetic. Not so. In fact, I think it is a simple, great way for everyone to see how their body responds to what they eat.

Some of you may already have a glucose meter and know how to test your blood sugar. Others may want to get a meter at their local drugstore. The newer ones are easy to use and you can always ask your pharmacist to show you how. I like the ACCU-CHEK Aviva Blood Glucose Meter with Strips, which includes a few test strips (you may need extra).

Here is the protocol I recommend for testing:

- Measure your fasting blood sugar daily, first thing in the morning before breakfast. Ideally your fasting blood sugar should be between 70 and 80 mg/dL.
- Measure your blood sugar two hours after breakfast and two hours after dinner. Ideally your two-hour sugars should never go over 120 mg/dL. If they go over 140 mg/dL, you have pre-diabetes. If they

go over 200 mg/dL, you have type 2 diabetes. Technically this is after a 75-gram glucose load, but if they go this high on the plan you definitely have a problem. Pay attention to how they change depending on what you eat over the ten days.

Get Tested with Your Doctor

Part of what you're doing over these ten days is becoming an active partner in your health and weight loss plan, and that includes having a full understanding of your numbers and following them over time. I believe everyone should become empowered to learn about their bodies, interpret their test results, and use that information to track their progress. I strongly encourage you to consider getting basic lab tests done before and after the program. These would include the following:

- Insulin response test, which is like a two-hour glucose tolerance test, but it measures insulin as well as glucose three times: after fasting, and one and two hours after a 75-gram glucose drink.
- Hemoglobin A1c, which measures your average blood sugar over the last six weeks. Anything over 5.5 percent is considered elevated, and over 6.0 percent is diabetes.

The lab tests above can be done through your doctor and at most hospitals or laboratories, or ordered yourself through personal testing companies such as SaveOnLabs (www.saveonlabs.com). For more information and detailed explanations for each of these tests, go to www.10daydetox .com/tools.

- NMR lipid (cholesterol) profile, which measures LDL, HDL, and triglycerides, as well as the particle number and, importantly, the particle size of each type of cholesterol and triglycerides. Diabesity causes you to have many small dangerous LDL and HDL cholesterol particles. This is a newer test, but I would demand it from your doctor, because the typical cholesterol tests done by most labs and doctors are out of date. This test can be obtained only through LabCorp or LipoScience.

Keep a record of your initial results and then track your progress as I've outlined above. You can do this with a simple pen and paper, or you use the online tools at www.10daydetox.com/tools for tracking all your scores, measurements, and vital stats, as well as your daily experiences and feelings through the detox journal.

3

Why Cook?

With our busy lives, so many of us shy away from cooking. Between our never-ending to-do lists, demanding jobs, busy children's schedules, and perhaps less-than-stellar skills in the kitchen, cooking seems to slide down the list of priorities. But when you consider all of the benefits of making a meal, you'll be inspired to channel your inner chef. Cooking a meal for yourself, a family member, or a friend is an act of love. It's a chance to strengthen bonds, teach important life-extending skills to our children, and enrich and nourish our bodies and our souls. The food industry wants us to believe that cooking is difficult, time consuming, inconvenient, and expensive, but meals need not be complicated or time consuming to be delicious and satisfying. The science is clear. You can eat well for less money by making simple, whole, fresh food. In fact, a simple dinner for a family of four consisting of roast chicken, vegetables, and salad can cost about half of what dinner out at McDonald's would cost.

I once visited an obese sick family who had never cooked. They lived on food stamps and disability. With one simple cooking lesson and a guide from the Environmental Working Group called "Good Food on a Tight Budget," they started cooking. In the first year, the mother lost over 100 pounds, the father lost 45 pounds, and their teenage son lost 40 pounds. Unfortunately, the son has since gained the weight back because the only jobs for teenagers in the food desert where they live are at a fast food chain. It's like sending an alcoholic to work in a bar! These days over 50 percent of meals are consumed outside the home, but it's my goal to get you to reconnect with your kitchen and the bounty of benefits it offers.

The reasons are simple. With today's toxic food environment—the slick combination of sugar, salt, and fat that's pumped into a wide range of packaged food—our genes (and our jeans) are overwhelmed. Our taste buds have been assaulted and our tongues and brains adapt by craving even more of these toxins. However, our hormones and biochemical pathways haven't adapted to this style of eating. The result is that nearly 70 percent of Americans are overweight, and obesity rates in the United States are expected to top 42 percent by the end of the next decade (up from only 13 percent in 1960).

Today one in two Americans has either pre-diabetes or diabetes. In less than a decade the rate of pre-diabetes or diabetes in teenagers has risen from 9 percent to 23 percent. Perhaps even more shocking, 37 percent of kids at a normal weight have pre-diabetes and one or more cardiovascular risk factors such as high blood pressure, high cholesterol, or high blood sugar, because even though overly processed food doesn't necessarily make you fat, it can make you sick. In addition to raising the risk for chronic, life-threatening diseases, the sad truth is that obese children will earn less, suffer more, and die younger.

But all of this can be reversed, and the cure lies in your kitchen. It also lies in your supermarket, not just with the fresh foods in the produce aisle, but also with some of the packaged foods that are tucked away in the middle. Healthy foods such as nuts and nut butters and nondairy milks are hidden gems in the middle aisles of the store. There are even brands making healthy packaged meals using quality ingredients from real, whole food—for those nights when cooking truly is out of the question. Some companies, such as Luvo (www.luvoinc.com), have created high-quality, delicious, affordable, and healthy frozen meals.

By purchasing these foods, you're going to transform yourself, but you're also helping to transform the food industry one small choice at a time. The problems are global, but the solution is as local as your fork! The movement is already under way, being driven by those of us who are fed up with Big Food poisoning our taste buds and our bodies. You have the power to join the movement, and it doesn't take a picket line or even a huge pocketbook. All it takes is voting with your wallet at the grocery store.

It's time for a revolution. Cooking real food is a revolutionary act. Without kitchen skills, we have lost the means to care for ourselves. Our children will grow up without these survival tactics, and their children will face the same fate—not being able to identify common fruits and vegetables, and not realizing where food comes from. I urge you to reconsider whatever notions you have about cooking—that it costs too much, that it's too hard, that it takes too long. The recipes within this cookbook are designed to challenge these myths, to reunite you with real food, and to delight your taste buds while nourishing your body. As an added bonus, you may find, as I do, that cooking can be fun and relaxing.

THE FAMILY KITCHEN

There is a reason why today's modern kitchens are open and inviting: People love to gather in the kitchen. It's the place for nourishing your body and your relationships. It's a space in which to bond with your children while teaching them valuable life skills.

Sadly, today's overscheduled families have a difficult time slowing down and tapping into this sacred space and all the wonders it has to offer. If this sounds familiar, I encourage you to reclaim your kitchen and your family time. Look carefully at your days and examine where you spend your time. Are you watching TV at night? Spending an hour on Facebook and Instagram? Most Americans spend more time watching someone cook on television than actually cooking. After close consideration, you may find that you can reorganize your to-do list, revisit your viewing habits, shut off your computer, and recover your precious time.

What we need is a lifestyle that makes cooking easy, inviting, and fun. And whether you're preparing food together or passing it around the family table, dinner is a wonderful time to reconnect, get the day's download, share laughs, and discuss important events. Start your new ritual by making your kitchen as warm and inviting as possible. Create a family playlist that puts everyone in a good mood. Invest in terrific lighting. Change your curtains. Open your windows. Put stools by the counter, or pillows on your chairs. Make the kitchen a place you and your family *want* to gather.

Once you set up the environment for success, let the fun begin! If you're new to cooking or your skills have gotten rusty, don't aim for perfection with your first recipe—experiment and practice. Start with one of my more basic recipes, with only a few ingredients, and work your way up to something more complex. Enlist help from family members—drag your kids away from their video games and ask them to measure ingredients, pull food from the fridge, or even chop veggies if they're ready to take on this task. Decide on meals together to get everyone excited about what's in store.

I encourage you to start your own family traditions around cooking and enjoying meals together. One of my favorite things to do with my kids is to hang out in the kitchen, chopping vegetables, telling stories, catching up, cooking, and anticipating sharing a great meal together. Once you get in the habit of nourishing your family life in this way, you'll never want to return to solo dining out of plastic containers and take-out boxes.

DINNER CONVERSATIONS: CREATING MAGIC AT MEALTIME

Want to make a great meal even better? Share it over an inspired dinner conversation.

Life coach Lauren Zander (cofounder of the Handel Group and creator of the Handel Method) has a fantastic mealtime tradition I'd like to share. She calls it "Creating a Conversation."

It works like this: At the start of the meal, your family or dinner guests suggest a potential question to be answered by each person at the table.

Everyone must agree on the question. Once a question is decided upon, everyone at the table *must* answer. The magic happens as everyone shares about themselves and connects with one another. You will get to know your family and friends on a deeper level.

To help you get started, here's a list of some of our favorite dinner conversations:

- What's your favorite thing about the person sitting to your right? Why?
- How would you describe the person on your left to someone who had never met them before?
- What's your favorite thing about the current season (winter, spring, summer, or fall)? What makes it special to you? What's your best memory from this season?
- What's something you can confess that nobody at the table knows about you?
- If you could pick any career in the world, regardless of ability or age, what would it be? Why?
- Dream up a new career for everyone at the table—if you could pick any job in the world for them, what would it be? Why?
- What's a city, town, or country you've never seen that you'd like to visit? Why?
- What's your very first memory of life?
- Tell the story of your first true love. Who was it? How old were you? What happened? Do you know anything about where they are right now?
- If the house was on fire and you could save just one of your possessions, what would it be? Why?
- If you could change one thing about yourself, what would it be? Why?
- What's the most embarrassing thing that has ever happened to you? What did you learn from it?
- If you could give the person to your left a superpower, what would it be? Why?

- What's something you saw, heard, or experienced this week that touched you?
- Tell a story of someone you deeply loved. Let us know what made that person special.
- What do you love most about your life? Why?
- What's something you do that makes you feel powerful? Why?
- Everyone has their own magic gift (e.g., finding a parking spot, intuitively knowing when someone important to you is sad or having a hard time). What's your magic gift?
- Imagine something you really want to achieve in your life. How will you achieve this?
- If you could invite a historical figure to dinner tonight, who would it be? Why? What would you ask him or her?
- If you could date anyone on earth, past or present, who would it be? Why?
- If you were stranded on a desert island for a year and could pick three CDs and one book, or three books and one CD, what would you choose?
- If you had unlimited funds and a month off starting tomorrow, what would you do?
- What is your slogan/theme song/motto for living life? Explain why, and how it impacts your life.
- What three things are guaranteed to make you smile?
- What song do you love to sing at the top of your lungs? What makes you love it?
- Name something you're scared of but would love to find the guts to do.
- What moment in life gave you goose bumps and why?
- What's something you tried to do but failed? What did you learn by failing?
- Make a wish for each person at the table for something you'd like to see them accomplish this year.
- If you could combine three people on earth (alive or dead, famous or not) to be your perfect mate, who would they be? Why?

I would love to hear from you about your favorite dinner conversation. You can post your favorite conversation-starting questions at www.10daydetox.com/tools.

And, if you want more help turning your dreams into reality, then please visit Coach Lauren's website (www.handelgroup.com) to learn more about how she and her team can help you dream big.

NUTRITION 101: WHAT WE NEVER LEARNED IN SCHOOL

The foundation of your diet should be high-quality protein, fats, and nonstarchy vegetables that don't spike blood sugar or insulin. The reasons are simple: These are the types of foods that not only detoxify your body, reignite your metabolism, calm body-wide inflammation, and crush cravings, but also fill you up. Remember it is very hard to control *how much* you eat, but easy to control *what* you eat. It is the quality of the food and the composition of your meal that matters most in reversing weight gain and creating health.

When you eat the right combination of foods, you can eat until you're gently satisfied without focusing on calories or portion sizes, and excess weight will come off naturally. But since calories have been the focus of conversations around weight loss and health for so long, I'll put it this way: If you eat four Twizzlers—a small amount by most standards—you would consume about 160 calories, and it's unlikely they would put a dent in your hunger. However, for those same 160 calories, you could have a heaping spoonful of almond butter and a practically endless supply of cherry tomatoes, jicama, and celery. I think you'll agree which is the more filling option. Not only that, a snack of nuts helps stabilize your blood sugar and provides you with lots of vitamins, minerals, and phytochemicals—health-protecting substances that ward off diseases such as type 2 diabetes, heart disease, and Alzheimer's disease. The Twizzlers? They have the opposite effect.

Snack foods such as Twizzlers and other hyperprocessed fare are high on the glycemic index (GI). This is a measure of how quickly a carbohydrate raises your blood sugar level. The index is measured on a scale of

0 to 100, with glucose (a form of simple sugar) having a value of 100. Higher numbers mean that a food causes a sharper rise in blood sugar. It's easy to see why candy would be considered a fast-acting carbohydrate, but you may be surprised to learn that any white flour—white rice, white bread, refined cereals, and even some whole-grain breads—convert to simple sugars in your body quite rapidly. In fact, bread has a higher GI than table sugar or sucrose; 2 slices of whole-wheat bread will raise your blood sugar more than 2 tablespoons of table sugar. On the other hand, nonstarchy vegetables, protein, nuts, seeds, and good fats raise blood sugar levels slowly.

While the glycemic index can be a helpful tool, it doesn't take into account what the rest of your meal looks like, or even how your food is cooked. All of this can impact your blood sugar levels. The best approach to meals is to combine slow-acting carbohydrates—those veggies listed in the produce section on page 41—with lean proteins and healthy fats. In fact, the 10-Day Detox Diet is a high-carb diet—because nonstarchy vegetables, fruits, and even nuts and seeds are all carbs—so it might be more accurate to call it a right-carb diet. You can shift the composition of your diet to help balance your blood sugar, and this will speed up your metabolism, activate burning of belly fat, and cut hunger and cravings. The goal, whether you're eating in your family's dining room, at your work cafeteria, or in a fine restaurant, is to always build your meal from these three types of foods. These three basics—quality proteins, healthy fats, and nonstarchy veggies—can be mixed and matched in any number of ways, so you'll never tire of your options. Have a miso-glazed salmon fillet with bok choy sautéed in avocado oil. Enjoy a spicy chicken breast over a chopped salad with a drizzle of fine olive oil. Dig into a juicy steak served with roasted broccoli and cauliflower. At every meal, you can enjoy a variety of foods, flavors, and textures so you'll never be bored.

Herbs, spices, and seasonings kick your cuisine, and your health, up a notch. Think of your spice cupboard as your new medicine cabinet and stock it with every imaginable seasoning. By flavoring your food liberally, you're not only keeping your taste buds happy, but you're also adding loads of phytonutrients to your meal. Cinnamon, cumin, turmeric, and cayenne pepper—to name just a few—have properties that stabilize blood sugar, quell inflammation, and boost metabolism. Different spices and seasonings have different benefits, which is why I always have lots of these gems on hand. Just be sure to use up your spices often and keep them sealed tightly in jars, as they become less potent with time.

The 10-Day Detox Diet Frozen Meals

Even those of us with the best intentions don't always have time to shop and cook. That's why the chefs at Luvo and I have collaborated on Luvo's Blood Sugar Solution 10-Day Detox Meals. You can get fully prepared, ready-to-heat meals — such as Thai Style Chicken Curry, Salmon Poblano, and Rosemary Garlic Beef — delivered to your home to help you stick to the diet.

Just like all Luvo entrées, this menu is phytonutrient rich. We use herbs, spices, and seasonings to create incredible flavors while promoting health. Luvo meals are naturally nutrient-rich, delicious, and not dependent on artificial flavors. They're also high in fiber and contain healthy fats and nutrients commonly missing from the typical American diet.

To learn more or to order the meals, go to luvoinc.com/10-day-detox.

4

Creating a Healing Kitchen

It's quite likely that your kitchen has been held hostage by the food industry. No doubt your cupboards and pantry are filled with ultra-processed fare. Now's your chance to escape these shackles and transform your kitchen into a place of wellness. If you make your kitchen a safe zone, with only foods that nourish rather than harm, then you will automatically make the right choices when it comes time to eat.

Ideally, you're starting the transformation at least two days before you begin your detox. This will give you enough time to clean out your cupboards and fridge, and restock with healing fare.

Start by setting aside at least an hour to scour and purge your pantry, fridge, and freezer. This is your time to do some detective work, read food labels, and dump anything that got you to this food-addicted, toxic state to begin with.

Ideally, your kitchen will mostly showcase foods without labels. Fresh avocados, blueberries, tomatoes, and kiwis don't come in packages and are label-free. But other foods, including nuts, nut butters, almond milk, canned fish, and frozen veggies—foods that I encourage you to eat—do come in packages. Further, once you enter the transition phase, you will be choosing gluten-free grains and other foods that are also minimally processed. It's clear that not *all* packages are bad—and that is why it is so important to get the hang of reading a nutrition facts panel and ingredients list. There is a short learning curve, but once you get the hang of it you will easily spot trouble. Follow these rules when you purchase packaged foods (i.e., anything with a nutrition label):

- **Beware of foods with health claims** on the packaging—such as "reduced sugar" or "no trans fat." These claims usually signal a marketing ploy to make you think the foods are good for you when they're really just pretenders. Things such as sports beverages, energy bars, and even multigrain breads (which often contain high-fructose corn syrup) fall into this category.

- **Focus on the ingredients list.** Remember that the most abundant ingredient is always listed first; the others follow in descending order by weight.

- **Choose foods with fewer than five ingredients** listed, and all things you recognize and know are real food—for example: "tomatoes, water, salt."

- **Buy only packaged foods with ingredients you can pronounce or recognize.** Need to buy something with more than five ingredients? The exception is if they are all whole-food, real ingredients such as spices. The main distinction is that the recipes don't call for things such as "maltodextrin" or "autolyzed yeast extract" or "high-fructose corn syrup." I don't stock these items in my kitchen, and neither should you. Bottom line: You should not eat packaged foods that contain ingredients you wouldn't have in your own kitchen.

- **Be aware that food manufacturers don't have to list ingredients that appear in trace amounts.** These trace ingredients could trip you up in your detox and lifelong quest for eating simple, healthy food. So always be vigilant when selecting multi-ingredient packaged foods. Stick with organic brands, or simple products, or those that declare themselves as gluten- or dairy-free.

- **Avoid these ingredients at all costs** during the 10-Day Detox Diet:
  - **Sugar.** You have to watch for all forms of sugar, not just the word "sugar." There are 257 forms of sugar, most made from corn, with names that you wouldn't recognize, such as maltodextrin and xanthan gum. There are many aliases to watch out for—including organic cane juice, honey, agave, maple syrup,

cane syrup, or molasses. And, look carefully at condiments such as salad dressing, barbecue sauce, or ketchup: There may be up to 33 teaspoons of sugar—often in the form of high-fructose corn syrup—in the average bottle of ketchup (about 1 teaspoon of sugar for every tablespoon of ketchup!). When transitioning off the detox, consider adding sugar back into your diet only as a special treat—to be enjoyed occasionally in small amounts.

- **Other sweeteners** (aspartame, NutraSweet, Splenda, sucralose, and sugar alcohols—any word that ends with "ol," such as xylitol or sorbitol). Stevia may be better than aspartame but only in the form of a whole-plant extract, not Pure Via or Truvia, which are made by Pepsi and Coke and are chemical extracts of stevia. Use it sparingly. A new noncaloric sweetener that comes from monk fruit (also called *luo han guo*) is rich in antioxidants and can also be used in small amounts. But remember, any sweetener can make you hungry, lower your metabolism, create gas, store belly fat, and even change your gut bacteria from those that make you thin to those that make you fat. So it's best to stay away from sweeteners altogether.

- **Bad fats.** Scour labels for the words "hydrogenated fat," just another name for trans fat. As you probably know, the Food and Drug Administration (FDA) has finally declared trans fats not suitable for human consumption. Yet the government has given food companies years to "reformulate" their products, so most processed or packaged foods still contain trans fats...and when there are trace amounts, they are not required to list them. So stay away from industrial, manufactured foodlike substances and science projects.

- **Preservatives, additives, colorings, natural flavorings.** Watch for ingredients you don't recognize or can't pronounce, or that are in Latin. Most of you know that MSG (monosodium glutamate) is a popular taste enhancer, but did you know that it is a brain toxin that causes compulsive overeating and spikes insulin? Knowing this sure makes it easier to avoid this ingredient, doesn't it?

- □ **Dairy.** Because milk is one of the eight most common food allergens, manufacturers are required to clearly identify it on a food label. But casein, the offending protein in dairy, can be found in mayonnaise, chocolate, and "natural" flavors. So be sure to watch for it on the ingredients list.
- □ **Gluten.** Gluten is one of the most common triggers of inflammation in the body and increases cravings and weight gain. It can be lurking in soba noodles, tamari, miso, seasonings, and stock, so look for "gluten-free" listings for these ingredients. But remember, gluten-free cookies are still cookies, and probably contain sugar and other things your body doesn't need.
- □ **Alcohol and caffeine.**
- ■ **Beware the "Nutrition Facts"** section of the label. Here's why:
  - □ **Not the whole story.** A typical nutrition facts label will give you quick stats on cholesterol, fat, carbohydrate, protein, and other nutrients. But, for example, it doesn't differentiate between healthy omega-3 fats and inflammatory omega-6 fats. You can't tell if the quickly absorbed carbs are the bad kind that spike blood sugar or slow-burning, "smart" carbohydrates.
  - □ **The "chemical soup" is not on the label.** The "nutrition facts" can't tell you if your food is laced with chemical preservatives, fillers, additives, hormones, antibiotics, pesticides, fertilizers, gluten, dairy, artificial sweeteners, synthetic vitamins, food dyes, and other toxic junk typically present in processed foods. That's why we emphasize paying more attention to the ingredients list and not spending too much time on the nutrition facts label.
  - □ **Focus on fiber, sugar, and protein per serving.** These three facts will help you discern whether the food can help regulate your blood sugars or send them skyrocketing.
    - ▪ Keep total sugars less than 8 grams per meal.
    - ▪ Aim to include at least 5 to 10 grams of fiber with every meal.
    - ▪ Aim for a minimum of 10 grams of protein with every meal, but up to 30 or 40 grams is fine. Include protein with every

meal because it keeps your blood sugars stable, prevents cravings, and builds fat-blasting muscle. For more information on what amount of protein and nutrition is appropriate for you, please visit my online nutrition team at www.10daydetox .com/tools.

☐ **Serving size.** Look at this carefully to determine whether this is your "typical" portion, as labels can be deceiving. For example, a 20-ounce soda says "2.5 servings," but do you usually share your soda with 1.5 other people? All of the stats on the panel are related to serving size, so once you determine how much you eat, you can figure out how much of each nutrient you'll be getting.

☐ **Fats** are broken down by type. On most labels you will find total fat, saturated fat, and trans fat. Some labels of foods rich in fat (oil, for example) will also tell you how much monounsaturated and polyunsaturated fats you are getting. If your label shows only the former three, you can subtract the saturated and trans fat from the total fat content in order to know how many grams of mono- and polyunsaturated fats you are getting. Monounsaturated and omega-3 polyunsaturated fats should dominate this category. Saturated fats are turning out not to be the bad guys we thought they were. While they do raise LDL, they also increase HDL and good fluffy cholesterol particles. In fact, in a recent review of 72 studies, there was no correlation between fat—even saturated fat—and heart disease. You want to look for zero trans fats. But be careful: If a serving has less than 0.5 gram of trans fat, the nutrition facts label can legally say "zero trans fats." Cool Whip, for instance, says it contains zero trans fats, but the three main ingredients are water, hydrogenated vegetable oil (another term for trans fats), and high-fructose corn syrup.

☐ **Total carbohydrates** include the amount of sugar (whether naturally occurring or added during processing) as well as fiber. This gives you a picture of how the food will impact your blood sugar. Think of fiber as the drain stopper of your stomach. Fiber slows the rate at which sugar from your food enters your bloodstream from your intestines. So, the more fiber a food contains, the slower your blood sugar will rise upon eating it. If you don't currently eat a high-fiber diet, start adding fiber slowly so that you don't cause any digestive distress. Your ultimate goal should be to consume around 50 grams daily. That may sound like a lot, but if you eat according to the guidelines outlined in this book, you will have no problem achieving that. Remember that foods that are naturally low in sugar (less than 10 grams) and high in fiber (more than 5 grams) are slow-acting carbohydrates, the kind you want.

- **Fiber** is one of the main factors that determine how slowly (or quickly) a carbohydrate enters your bloodstream. Most of the packaged foods you'll be eating—such as nuts and frozen vegetables—are naturally rich in fiber. Some packaged foods, however, have added fibers. One type of fiber is called resistant starch because it escapes digestion in your small intestine. The fact is, you don't know what you are getting when you see this, and for all you know it could be sawdust! (Some bread makers actually use sawdust as a resistant starch to lower the net carbs of the bread.) Putting sawdust in food doesn't make it healthy; eating real forms of fiber such as vegetables, seeds, and nuts is healthy. Stay away from any type of fiber that is not naturally a part of your food. In fact, for the most part, if you see a fiber in the ingredients list, you know this product is better for the company's marketing department than your body! There are many ways to tell if a food product is good or lousy. If a manufacturer is bragging about the fiber content of a certain food, there's a good chance that fiber has been added in the form of inulin (also known as oligofructose or chicory root fiber), polydextrose, resistant starch, or wheat dextrin. Always scan the ingredients list to look for these terms and avoid foods made with them. Stick with whole-food fiber, not sawdust or engineered forms of fiber.
- **Cholesterol** in foods is not the problem we once thought it was. There is little correlation between dietary cholesterol and blood

cholesterol, and little reason to worry about this number on food labels. Surprising but true.

☐ **Sodium** is abundant in packaged foods. As much as 70 percent of the sodium in your diet could be coming from packaged food sold in your supermarket. Companies add sodium to give packaged foods flavor, but fresh foods don't need much salt to taste fabulous. When you eat whole foods, you naturally get the right amount of sodium your body needs. By following my program, you will easily cut down on and normalize your sodium intake. Current dietary guidelines suggest to keep sodium intake under 2,300 milligrams. Yet, new research shows that the lowest risk of mortality comes from an intake of 3,000 to 6,000 milligrams per day. Interestingly, Japanese people consume an average of 4,500 milligrams of sodium per day and have one of the highest life expectancies in the world, with low cardiovascular risk. What does all this mean? Sodium itself is not the culprit, but an unhealthy diet full of processed foods, inflammatory fats, and refined carbohydrates is. When you don't include fresh, real food—namely, potassium-rich vegetables and low-glycemic fruits—you increase your sodium-to-potassium ratio. Because potassium helps you excrete fluid, it helps to relieve the pressure in your circulatory system. If you consume too much sodium, as is the case when you eat a processed foods–based diet, your blood pressure may rise, especially if you have diabesity. The goal is to include plenty of potassium-rich foods and crowd out the sodium-rich processed junk. When you cook meals at home with these recipes you will learn how to add the right amount and type of salt to flavor your food and nourish your body. Play around with adding real flavor to your meals by using tasty seasonings such as curry powder, chile peppers, rosemary, sage, and cinnamon. The less salt you add, the less you will want, as your taste buds will adapt to your new eating habits.

☐ **Protein** is your secret weapon to success on this program because it reduces insulin spikes and keeps you feeling satisfied long after you've eaten. Each protein is made of specific amino acids. Amino acids are the building blocks of protein and are either essential or nonessential. Essential amino acids cannot be produced in the body and need to be consumed through diet, while nonessential amino acids can be produced in the body from other sources of carbohydrates or proteins. When we consume animal protein or soy protein, we ensure that our body receives complete, high-biological-value protein. This is important for detoxifying and getting and maintaining health. Remember that diversity is the key to nutrition, so eat a variety of whole foods to meet your protein needs. Opt for protein sources such as high-quality meat, clean fish, poultry, omega 3–enriched eggs, tofu, and nuts.

□ **Vitamins and minerals** are listed at the bottom of the nutrition facts panel, but eyeball these with caution. Sometimes junk foods are fortified with nutrients to enhance their appeal. For example, B vitamins are added to foods to "enrich" them, but that is only because they are impoverished in the first place. Obviously, a food put together from various artificial ingredients won't naturally contain the valuable nutrients you would get if you just ate the real thing. Take vitamin water, for example. It is a farce, a brilliant marketing ploy for one more type of sugar water sold by Coke. We all know that water doesn't naturally contain vitamins! And candy, too—do you really think gummy bears have naturally occurring vitamin C? Look at this part of the food panel carefully and you'll be able to sort out good food from junk food.

■ **Stay away from "foodlike substances."** These are things that, through processing, no longer resemble the real food in its true form. Veggie burgers made with soy protein isolates—a cheap form of processed soy—are a hijacked version of soy in its whole form (for example, tofu).

Knowing what to avoid is important. However, you are probably wondering about everything that is in your pantry and refrigerator right now. What's okay and not okay to use during the detox? What should I avoid and then safely reintroduce? Here's a general guide to the items that should be tossed out permanently or put aside for the next ten days.

ITEMS THAT NEED TO GO PERMANENTLY:

- Highly refined cooking oils such as corn and soy.
- Fried foods you may have stored in your freezer.
- Margarine or shortening, which contain those dreaded hydrogenated fats we discussed earlier.

ITEMS THAT SHOULD BE AVOIDED FOR THE NEXT TEN DAYS (find a spot for them where they are out of sight, as you may choose to reintroduce these in your transition phase):

- All gluten-containing products (including whole-grain versions), such as pasta, bread, and cereal.
- All grains (including gluten-free versions), such as quinoa and rice.
- All dairy products (including but not limited to butter, milk, yogurt, and cheese — from any animal).
- All beans (including chickpeas, lentils, and even peanuts, which are actually beans).
- Any prepared food that was made in your local store or by a small manufacturer. It's best to steer clear of premade foods altogether because certain items might be left off the ingredients list due to FDA labeling guidelines.
- All alcohol, as it is simply sugar in a different form, and it impairs impulse control so you're more likely to eat more — and to do so mindlessly. It also has more calories per gram than sugar (7 calories compared to 4 calories), provokes a leaky gut, and inflames your liver. While it is not all about the calories, if you have one glass of wine a day at 110 calories, over the course of a year that can add up to 11 pounds of weight gain.
- Caffeine. Some say caffeine speeds up metabolism or the rate of calorie burning, called *thermogenesis*. But so do spicy jalapeños or cayenne pepper. Caffeine is hidden in many soft drinks and energy

drinks because it is addictive, so you consume more of the sugary drinks. Caffeine also increases hunger.

Now that you've cleaned out your kitchen, you will automatically steer clear of the toxic foods that cause addiction, weight problems, and health struggles. Consider yourself liberated!

STOCKING YOUR KITCHEN WITH WHAT YOU *CAN* EAT — MY GUIDE TO LIVING CLEAN AND GREEN

Now that there's all that room in your fridge and cabinets, let's have some fun filling them up with real, fresh food. This is where we begin to discover all the amazing new options you have. Perhaps it's been a while since you explored the produce section of your grocery store or visited a farmers' market. Maybe you're unfamiliar with the bounty of fresh vegetables that you can use as the basis for many meals at the foundation of this program. The key to success is a well-stocked kitchen, which allows you to whip up a meal on even the busiest of days.

I am proud to be on the board of directors for the Environmental Working Group (EWG) because what we do to our bodies we do to the planet, and what we do to the planet we do to our bodies. The link between environmental toxins and chronic disease is now clear. We know that pesticides and other industrial chemicals cause obesity and type 2 diabetes. There is a new word for these compounds: *obesogens*. When we are toxic, we feel lousy, gain unwanted pounds, and have trouble losing them. Toxins disrupt the hormones that regulate our metabolism.

The recipes in this book will help you live clean and green by using foods that contain special phytochemicals that increase your body's capacity for detoxification and balance your blood sugar. They are designed to put your medicine on the end of your fork.

Here are some of the fresh and pantry food items you should always have on hand.

Produce

Fresh vegetables and fruits make up half of all of my meals. But before we go crazy buying just any produce, I'd like to talk a little bit about making the right selections. Agricultural chemical inputs such as pesticides and fertilizers leave a residue, which we as consumers absorb. Because these chemicals are fat-soluble, they become stored in our fat cells. Our bodies recognize these toxins as foreign, prompting an inflammatory response. Once our exposure surpasses our threshold, we become sick and fat.

When you can, avoid the most pesticide-contaminated fruits and vegetables. The EWG annually reviews conventional vegetables and fruits and publishes a list of those with the lowest and highest toxic load. EWG understands that we have a right to know which foods are safe and which we need to be concerned about. They provide many resources for consumers, including their Shopper's Guide, which helps consumers opt out of the produce posing the highest risk while saving their food dollars for the safer choices. For an easier reference, check out their "Dirty Dozen" and "Clean Fifteen" lists featuring the most- and least-contaminated options in the conventional food supply. Of course, you can still buy items from the "Dirty Dozen" list, but they should be organic. As of the date of publication of this book, these are featured below. To make the most informed choices for you and your loved ones, visit EWG's website at www.ewg.org for the most updated lists.

THE DIRTY DOZEN:

1. Apples
2. Strawberries
3. Grapes
4. Celery
5. Peaches
6. Spinach
7. Sweet bell peppers
8. Imported nectarines
9. Cucumbers

10. Cherry tomatoes
11. Imported snap peas
12. Potatoes

THE CLEAN FIFTEEN:

1. Avocados
2. Sweet corn
3. Pineapples
4. Cabbage
5. Frozen sweet peas
6. Onions
7. Asparagus
8. Mangoes
9. Papayas
10. Kiwis
11. Eggplant
12. Grapefruit
13. Cantaloupe
14. Cauliflower
15. Sweet potatoes

WHAT TO STOCK UP ON

- When possible, choose organic, seasonal, local produce. Be sure to check out your local farmers' market or community-supported agriculture (CSA) group. You can find the one closest to you at www.localharvest.org.
- For those living in colder climates, you can find organic versions of your favorite fruits and vegetables in the freezer section. Always make sure you're buying unseasoned or unsweetened varieties.
- Nonstarchy veggies are freebies—eat as many as you like! A limited selection of fruits are included on this plan because most fruits increase your insulin levels. I have included those fruits that support you with the right vitamins, minerals, and antioxidants. Following is a list of low-GI, low-sugar vegetables and fruits you can eat while on this

program. Many of them are incorporated into the delicious recipes in the pages ahead. If you have a few favorites that appear on this list but don't appear in the recipes, feel free to substitute them at any time.

- Artichokes
- Arugula
- Asparagus
- Avocados
- Bean sprouts
- Beet greens
- Bell peppers
- Blueberries
- Broccoli
- Brussels sprouts
- Cabbage
- Cauliflower
- Celery
- Chives
- Collard greens
- Dandelion greens
- Eggplant
- Endive
- Fennel
- Fresh herbs
- Garlic
- Ginger
- Green beans
- Hearts of palm
- Jalapeños
- Kale
- Kiwis
- Lemons
- Lettuce
- Limes
- Mushrooms
- Mustard greens
- Onions
- Pomegranate seeds
- Radicchio
- Radishes
- Shallots
- Snap peas
- Snow peas
- Spinach
- Summer squash
- Swiss chard
- Tomatoes
- Turnip greens
- Watercress
- Zucchini

Fresh Meats and Proteins

What about meat, poultry, fish, and eggs? As best you can, limit your exposure to excessive hormones, antibiotics, and grain-fed meat. Select wild meat, grass-fed when possible, and organic poultry and eggs. Because we eat what the animal ate, we want our animal-based protein to have been fed the highest-quality diet. An animal fed its natural diet, typically grass and plants, contains fewer stress hormones, growth hormones, and antibiotics than a feedlot animal or industrially produced animal foods. By selecting higher-quality animal-based proteins, you can be sure you are getting healthier fats and leaner, cleaner protein.

When it comes to selecting poultry, the U.S. Department of Agriculture (USDA) mandates that all poultry be raised without the use of hormones. However, chicken producers must give medications to those birds that get sick before selling them. Therefore, always look for the terms "antibiotic-free" or "organic" when buying poultry to ensure you are truly getting a toxin-free product.

Get in the habit of keeping your fridge and freezer stocked with the items below:

- Grass-fed, hormone-free, or organic beef, lamb, and bison (buffalo) meat (refer to the Environmental Working Group's "Meat Eater's Guide" at www.ewg.org to choose meat that's good for you and good for the planet).
- Organic or antibiotic-free boneless, skinless chicken and turkey breasts and ground chicken and turkey.
- Wild or sustainably farmed low-mercury seafood such as clams, crab, flounder, herring, oyster, perch, pollock, salmon, sardines, shrimp, sole, squid, trout, and whitefish. Avoid fish that are high in mercury, such as tuna, swordfish, and Chilean sea bass. Go to the National Resources Defense Council website (www.nrdc.org) and download their Sustainable Seafood Guide to choosing the fish lowest in mercury.
- Organic omega 3–enriched eggs.
- Organic, whole forms of non-GMO (genetically modified organisms) soy food, such as tofu, tempeh, and gluten-free, low-sodium miso.

With these healthy pantry staples in your cooking arsenal, you'll be amazed at the delicious and nutritious dishes you can create. Cooking food that tastes great and nourishes your body doesn't need to break the bank, either—and that's why I stock my pantry with food from Thrive Market. See page 5 to learn how you can get a free two-month membership.

Healing Pantry Staples

The recipes in this book celebrate real, whole, fresh food. They are easily made in your kitchen yet taste as if they came from a restaurant. We live in a food desert, so our reliance on getting back into the kitchen to enjoy a meal that is both satisfying and healthy requires us to learn how to cook again. The following are some of the ingredients I use the most in my own kitchen :

- Extra-virgin olive oil
- Extra-virgin coconut butter/oil (at room temperature it is solid, but it melts into a liquid)
- Other healthy oils, such as walnut, sesame, grapeseed, flax, or avocado
- Nut butters (raw, if possible), such as almond, cashew, macadamia, or walnut
- Nuts, such as walnuts, almonds, pecans, and macadamias
- Seeds, such as hemp, chia, flax, pumpkin, and sesame
- Tahini (sesame seed paste)
- Full-fat unsweetened coconut milk
- Unsweetened hemp or almond milk
- Canned or jarred Kalamata olives
- Almond flour (also called almond meal)
- Arrowroot
- Apple cider vinegar
- Balsamic vinegar
- Gluten-free, low-sodium tamari
- Low-sodium vegetable or chicken stock
- Dijon mustard
- Sea salt
- Black peppercorns (for grinding)
- Dried herbs and spices, such as basil, cayenne pepper, chili powder, cinnamon, coriander, cumin, onion powder, oregano, paprika, parsley, rosemary, sage, thyme, turmeric

Some of the items listed above may be familiar to you and others not so much. Whether you are new to cooking or just to learning how to cook healthy options, I want to introduce you to some amazing ingredients that can enhance your meals and provide some variety:

Almond Flour

Made from blanched and finely ground almonds, almond flour (also known as almond meal) is a low-glycemic alternative to grain-based flours such as wheat flour. Use almond flour in place of gluten-based flours when making muffins, breads, or other baked goods.

Arrowroot

During the 10-Day Detox Diet, all grains, including corn, need to be omitted from your meal plan. Arrowroot is a corn-free, hypoallergenic alternative to cornstarch. Remember, corn in any form is still a grain and a potential allergen. Arrowroot is a useful culinary tool for your sauces or stews.

Chia Seeds

Chia seeds are one of the few vegetarian and vegan sources of omega-3 fatty acids. When they absorb water, they gel into a pudding-like substance that adds great texture to shakes, desserts, and cereals.

Coconut Aminos

If you are soy-intolerant, try using a little coconut aminos for that soy sauce flavor. It is made from the sap of the palm tree and imparts a slightly sweet aftertaste. Coconut aminos are rich in amino acids—the building blocks of protein.

Coconut Butter

I use coconut butter to add a silky texture and buttery flavor to morning shakes. It is made from whole coconut flesh, not just the oil. The butter provides fiber, protein, and nutrients to help keep you satisfied. Coconut butter can be found in most grocery stores near the other nut and seed butters.

Coconut Cream

When you remove excess water from coconut milk and strain it, you are left with a rich cream that is slightly sweet and full of healthy fat. It is a great alternative to dairy cream—a little bit goes a long way.

Coconut Flour

Coconut flour is a nutty, slightly sweet alternative to grain-based flours. Unlike wheat flour, coconut flour is not heavily refined, so most of its nutrition remains intact. Dried coconut meat is defatted and ground to a granular texture. It is useful in baked products and often found in grain-free cereals. High in fiber and very low in carbohydrates, it is a great tool in your detox kitchen.

Coconut Milk

The slightly sweet flavor of coconut milk makes it a healthy alternative to dairy milk. It is rich in saturated fat and healthy medium-chain triglycerides, which studies show boost metabolism and have other health benefits. You can buy whole-fat organic canned coconut milk and mix it with four cans of water to create your own coconut milk without sweeteners or stabilizers.

Coconut Oil

Coconut oil is extracted from the whole coconut, and unlike coconut butter, the oil does not contain fiber or protein. Studies have shown that coconut oil, used in sautés, shakes, sauces, or baking, helps improve blood sugar regulation, boosts immunity, and even increases the ratio of HDL to LDL cholesterol so you have more healthy lipids in your circulation. Look for whole-kernel, expeller-pressed coconut oil to get the most benefits.

Flaxseed Meal

Flaxseed meal is a nutrition powerhouse and a great vegetarian source of omega-3 fatty acids, lignans, and fiber. Add a tablespoon or two to shakes to add fiber and promote healthy elimination. Use freshly ground flax-seed meal when possible, and store it in your refrigerator.

Grapeseed Oil

Grapeseed oil is extracted from the seeds of grapes. It has a healthy fat profile of monounsaturated and polyunsaturated fats. I use it for higher-heat cooking and baking as it has a higher smoke point (the point at which an oil smokes and becomes rancid). Because it has a neutral flavor, you can use it as a healthier alternative to canola oil.

Hemp Protein Powder

Hemp protein powder is a hypoallergenic plant-based protein that can boost the protein content of your morning shakes or smoothies. Look for unsweetened protein powders. Sometimes hemp protein is combined with chia, rice, or pea proteins for a vegetarian or vegan protein blend with a smooth texture.

Hemp Seed

Hemp seed is an excellent complete protein as it contains all nine essential amino acids as well as essential fatty acids such as omega-3 fats. It has an earthy, nutty flavor, which balances the sweetness of berries in your morning shakes. Enjoy it in smoothies, nut and seed mixes, or even baked on chicken.

Kelp Noodles

Kelp noodles are made from the sea vegetable. They are simple to prepare, eaten raw, and low in carbohydrates. Their neutral flavor makes them fun to include in meals containing sauces such as curries or in broths such as miso soup.

Mayonnaise

Real mayo, made from omega 3–enriched eggs, is simple to make and adds an indulgence to your snacks and sauces. I've included a recipe (page 299) so you can avoid the unhealthy soybean oils, preservatives, and sugar in store-bought mayo.

Miso

Miso adds a deep, comforting element to dishes and intensifies the overall flavor. There are various kinds of miso, ranging from white and yellow, which tend to be mild, to red, brown, and even black miso. Generally, the deeper the color, the longer the miso has fermented and the stronger the taste. Mild miso tastes less salty, and stronger miso offers more of that umami, or savory, salty taste. Some miso pastes have been fermented with grains, especially gluten grains such as barley. Be sure to use miso that has only soybeans, water, and salt on the ingredients list. Brown miso, such as *hatcho,* is gluten-free and contains only fermented soybeans.

Mustard

Mustard, made from ground mustard seeds, is rich in antioxidants and other detox-friendly phytonutrients. Mustard is a lovely complement to any fish, chicken, or meat. It is also delicious in homemade dressings, marinades, and sauces.

Palm Shortening

Palm shortening, made from palm oil, is a great alternative to hydrogenated oils traditionally used in shortening. I like it because it has 0 trans fats and is gluten- and dairy-free. You'll find that it works well in baking because it has a neutral flavor and adds that tasty, fatty mouth feel you are used to enjoying in baked goods.

Sea Salt

When you eat real food and not overly salted processed food, you can use more salt. While seafood, meat, and some vegetables are naturally rich in sodium, you can still enjoy flavoring your meals with moderate quantities of real sea salt. Avoid table salt, which is refined and devoid of sulfur, zinc, iron, calcium, potassium, and magnesium, which naturally occur in sea salt.

Seaweed

Vegetables from the sea, such as dulse, wakame, nori, and kombu, are dense in minerals and vitamins such as potassium, calcium, iron, magnesium, iodine, and selenium. Use seaweed in salads, soups, and stews to add a hint of savory.

Shirataki Noodles

Traditionally made with konjac root, these low-glycemic noodles are gluten- (and guilt-) free.

Tamari

Look for gluten-free, low-sodium tamari for a healthier alternative to soy sauce.

Thai Fish Sauce

Fish sauce has a complex flavor that complements the sweet flavors of traditional Thai cooking. I love using a dash of fish sauce to impress dinner guests. It adds that wow factor that will leave your guests wondering how you learned to cook so well!

Replace This with That

For the next ten days, you're challenged with a radical change in the way you've been eating. My bet is that after the ten days are up, you'll want to stick to many of the principles of the basic plan. Once you get into the transition phase, you can start to gradually add in other foods, depending on how much weight you still need to lose and your personal health goals. I offer the following suggestions to help you adapt to this way of life, but feel free to get creative in the kitchen to find substitutions that help you stay on track.

INSTEAD OF	TRY
Fruit-flavored yogurt	Chia pudding
Pasta	Shirataki noodles
Mashed potatoes	Cauliflower mash
Rice	Cauliflower "rice"
Peanut butter	Almond or other nut butters
Potato chips, pretzels, tortilla chips	Nuts
Parmesan cheese	Nutritional yeast
Cornstarch	Arrowroot
Dairy milk	Unsweetened coconut milk or almond milk
Canned tuna	Canned wild salmon
Butter	Coconut oil or butter
Wheat flour	Almond flour or coconut flour
Bread, wraps, or buns	Bibb or romaine lettuce leaves
Milk chocolate	Raw cacao or 75% dark chocolate

5

Tips and Tools

Now that we have discussed the facts behind making the right choices, identified the good and the bad, and helped you restock your kitchen for success, I'd like to provide you with some quick tips to make the next ten days—and the rest of your life—a little easier. Change and transition are not easy, so hopefully the information on the next few pages will be useful.

KITCHEN TOOL ESSENTIALS

Would you set out to begin a DIY project without a hammer or other necessary equipment? Of course not! If you want to cook you need a well-stocked kitchen. I suggest you have the following tools on hand— they'll make cooking fast, simple, and fun.

- a set of good-quality knives
- two wooden cutting boards—one for animal products, another for fruits and vegetables
- an 8-inch and a 12-inch nonstick (non-Teflon) sauté pan
- an 8-quart stockpot
- a 2-quart and a 4-quart saucepan with lids
- an 11-inch-square nonstick (non-Teflon) stovetop griddle
- a Dutch oven
- a grill pan
- several rimmed baking sheets

- several square and/or rectangular baking dishes
- a food processor
- a blender
- an immersion blender
- an instant-read thermometer
- a coffee grinder for flaxseed and spices
- wire whisks
- spring tongs
- a fish spatula
- rubber spatulas
- a vegetable steaming rack or basket
- assorted measuring cups, metal for dry ingredients and glass for liquids
- assorted measuring spoons
- a citrus reamer
- Microplane graters/zesters in assorted sizes
- a food mill
- natural parchment paper and foil
- a timer
- sealable glass containers in various sizes for storing leftovers (plastic contains known hormone disruptors, which have been associated with insulin resistance and weight gain as well as female hormonal imbalance and thyroid disease)

SHORTCUTS AND TIME SAVERS

One question I am often asked is: How do I detox on a busy schedule? Trust me, it's easier than you think, but it does require a little planning. I find that when I invest that time, it pays off by keeping me healthy and eating well. In the end, it makes life a little easier, too. Here are some of my own recommended time savers:

- Cook once and eat twice by doubling the recipe and enjoying leftovers later in the week.

- Do as much prep work as possible the night before you plan to cook.
- Chop veggies ahead of time and store them in airtight containers, ready to be used in salads, stir-fries, and other recipes. Precut produce is also available at many markets, both in bags in the produce aisle and at the salad bar. Although it may be a bit more expensive, it drastically reduces prep work.
- Frozen vegetables (preferably organic) are a real time-saver—especially if you already have some in your freezer and can avoid the need for last-minute grocery store stops. Cascadian Farm, and some store brands, provide high-quality, organic frozen vegetables that were picked and flash-frozen at the peak of freshness.
- Choose fresh prewashed organic leafy greens, such as spinach, kale, arugula, and romaine lettuce.
- Make sauces and marinades and, if you're in the transition phase, cook brown rice and other whole grains in advance.
- Carefully chosen canned and jarred foods, such as vegetable or chicken stock, sardines, wild Alaskan salmon, artichoke hearts, and roasted red peppers, make it easy to toss together last-minute meals and enhance salads. Remember to choose low-sodium versions and read labels carefully to avoid gluten, dairy, sugars, and other unwanted ingredients.
- Choose two days during the week (Sunday and Wednesday seem to work well for many people) when you are going to spend a few extra hours in the kitchen, cooking and preparing as much as you can in advance. With all of your ingredients ready to go, a fresh home-cooked meal can be on the table in less time than it takes the take-out delivery to reach your home.

PLAN YOUR MEALS, SHOP, AND PREPARE FOOD IN ADVANCE

Let's face it: If you wait to decide what to eat until just before you leave for work or just after you get home in the evening, you may not have everything you need to put a meal on the table. Being caught off-guard while having a growling tummy could put you in danger of going off the program entirely and just grabbing what is available, quick, and easy—usually addictive, processed junk. That's where planning comes in. Take some time one day per week to sit down and plan your meals for the upcoming week, and make a shopping list. Go to the grocery store and purchase all of the ingredients for those recipes in advance. Make sure to stick a few frozen goodies in your cart—such as frozen produce or shrimp—which will come in handy as you work your way through the fresh food earlier in the week.

Remember, no matter how challenging the prep work seems at first, I promise you'll find that it gets easier and easier, and you'll be a whiz at planning meals in no time. You'll come to appreciate arriving home to a fridge filled with marinated meat and chopped veggies just waiting to be stir-fried.

I totally understand the instinct to order takeout when you're tired after a long day of work. But if you want to detoxify your body, calm the inflammation that's ravaging your system, balance your hormones, lose weight, and reverse diabesity, it's crucial to stick to the plan.

GOOD FOOD ON A TIGHT BUDGET

Relying on inexpensive, overly processed food is tempting, given our demanding lives and schedules, but the cost is actually much greater than it appears. Feasting on salt, fat, and sugar can lead to serious diseases that cost hundreds of dollars in doctor's visits and prescription drugs. We can become sick and sluggish, resulting in less productivity. We might have less patience for our loved ones and less energy to work or enjoy ourselves. Considering the real cost of cheap, processed food, you can't afford *not* to cook.

By now some of you might be wondering how to make this work on your budget. It helps to track all of your expenses for one week and see how much of what you spent went toward achieving your health goals. Right off the bat, you'll be able to spot recurring items and pricey habits that don't get you closer to your goals. For example, if you brew your own coffee each day instead of stopping at a coffee shop, you could save up to $1,500 a year. Do you order takeout for office lunches and Friday night dinners? You may be surprised to find that cooking your own food—even the high-quality food I'm talking about—can save you money. By reorganizing your budget and taking a look at other nonessential discretionary spending, you might create more funding for good food.

You can continue to save money even after you adjust your budget. I recommend getting a copy of "Good Food on a Tight Budget" by the Environmental Working Group (www.ewg.org) to learn what foods are good for you, good for the planet, and good for your wallet. Stick with simple ingredients and a handful of spices that you can use in many dishes, rather than expensive ingredients that you'd use less often. Shop at discount stores such as Trader Joe's or shopping clubs like Costco. Get fresh, local produce from a community-supported agriculture (CSA) group or farmers' market. Look at store circulars to see what's on sale, and shop private-label brands, many of which offer high-quality, organic staple items.

HEALTHY SNACKING

My version of detox doesn't involve juicing, fasting, or even hunger. You'll find that when you eat real, nutritious foods, you will be naturally satisfied. That said, if you go too long between meals or find that you are hungry outside of mealtimes, it helps to have a snack on hand.

For many, however, snacking has become reckless behavior, synonymous with eating a candy bar from a vending machine or nibbling through a bag of chips, a carton of cookies, or some other salty or sweet packaged item. Let's recast how you think about snacking so you can change your habits.

If you eat well and keep your blood sugar balanced according to the principles of the 10-Day Detox Diet, you probably won't need a snack. But sometimes you might. I view snacking as another occasion to flood your system with protective nutrients that quell hunger, quiet inflammation, and steady your blood sugar. Just as you do at meals, you should combine nonstarchy veggies with quality proteins and healthy fats for snacks. There are many flavorful ways to do this: Enjoy celery sticks with almond butter, a "mezze" plate with a variety of nuts and vegetables, a slice of natural deli meat (without nitrates, high-fructose corn syrup, or preservatives) spread with mashed avocado and wrapped around a romaine leaf, or a hardboiled egg with sliced red bell pepper. The beauty of the program is that you can be completely flexible once you get used to a few simple guidelines.

Although I don't believe in counting calories or policing portion sizes, your between-meal eating occasions should be smaller than your regular meals. Eat until you are comfortably satisfied, and there's a good chance you're eating the right amount. The key is to keep a variety of healthy snacks on hand so that you're not tempted to visit the vending machine when your stomach starts to growl.

6

How to Prepare Simple Meals

While you'll find that many of the recipes in this cookbook come together quickly and easily, I know that sometimes you are absolutely stuck for time. So, rather than go for the quick-and-dirty takeout option, check out this guide to putting together easy meals using just a few simple ingredients.

COOKING VEGETABLES

Steaming or sautéing veggies takes very little time—especially if you start with precut produce.

To Steam:

Pour 1 cup of water in the bottom of a saucepan and bring it to a boil over high heat. Place a steaming rack or basket over the boiling water.

Chop your veggies (or use precut ones), place them in the steaming rack, cover, and steam them for 4 to 8 minutes, depending on the vegetable and your desired level of tenderness. They should still be crunchy, as overcooked vegetables are mushy and less nutritious.

Add your favorite seasonings, drizzle with extra-virgin olive oil, and sprinkle with a little sea salt and freshly ground black pepper to taste. You can cook almost any vegetable this way, and both prep and cleanup are a breeze.

To Sauté:

Heat 1 tablespoon extra-virgin olive oil or other favorite oil, such as coconut oil, in a sauté pan over medium-high heat.

Chop your veggies (or use pre-cut ones) and drop them in. Sauté to your desired flavor and tenderness, 5 to 7 minutes.

Onions, garlic, and/or mushrooms are tasty additions to sautéed veggies. Not only do they make them more flavorful and fragrant, they also boost the phytonutrient content. You might want to sauté these first with a little salt before adding the chopped veggies. Add spices for extra flavor and healing power.

COOKING FISH, CHICKEN, AND MEAT

Fish, chicken, and meat are simple to prepare in a delicious and healthy way. Just grill, broil, or sauté, then season with olive oil, lemon juice, rosemary, garlic, ginger, and/or cilantro. Another easy flavor-enhancer and nutrient-booster is dairy-free pesto. See page 293 for a simple recipe—it will keep for months in your freezer, so you can make a big batch.

To Broil or Grill:

Preheat the broiler or grill. Sprinkle sea salt, freshly ground black pepper, and any other seasonings you like on your fish fillets or steaks; boneless, skinless chicken breasts; or lean cuts of meat. If you use spice blends, make sure they don't contain MSG and watch for salt (omit additional salt if it's already included in the spice blend).

Place the fish, chicken, or meat under the broiler or on the grill. Cook fish until it is tender and opaque throughout, 7 to 10 minutes, flipping it once. Chicken and meat will take longer, perhaps up to 15 minutes, depending on the thickness. Again, flip it once. The safest way to tell when chicken or meat is done is to check it with a meat thermometer. Chicken is ready when the thermometer registers 165°F; beef is ready at 145°; and pork and lamb are ready at 160°F. Fish is done once it starts to flake with a fork or when it registers 145°F. Be careful not to overcook your fish, chicken, or meat because it will become dry and tough.

To Sauté:

Sprinkle sea salt, freshly ground black pepper, and any other seasoning you like on your fish, chicken, or meat.

Heat 1 to 2 tablespoons extra-virgin olive oil in a sauté pan over medium-high heat. Place your fish, chicken, or meat in the pan. Turn fish or meat just once while cooking, but turn chicken often to avoid browning it too much on one side. Follow the same cooking times and temperatures as for broiling and grilling.

Once it is cooked, season your fish, chicken, or meat with additional sea salt, freshly ground black pepper, up to 1 tablespoon extra-virgin olive oil, and a few squirts of fresh lemon juice. You can also boost the flavor with fresh or dried herbs.

While the recipes in this book are designed to encourage you to cook real, delicious, and inspiring meals, you'll also find that you don't have to follow a recipe or spend hours in the kitchen to follow the program. Just stick to real foods prepared in simple ways and you'll notice that the pounds will come off, the cravings will disappear, and just about every aspect of your health will improve.

PART II

THE RECIPES

My mission is to help people rediscover the joy of eating real food. My personal and professional journey has led me to promote healthy eating. On this journey, I have met remarkable people and discovered amazing organizations. Together we are creating a movement of people who are passionate and ready to make a difference.

As my good friend Steve Sidwell, the founder of Luvo, says, "Food is the problem, but it is also the solution."

I am proud of my association with Luvo and my role as one of their ambassadors. We are working together to put into motion concrete solutions to the problem. Because we believe the solutions should be easy, I have collaborated with John Mitchell, Chief Innovation Officer at Luvo, to create all of the recipes in this book. Our mission is to reinvent "delicious." We want to show that delicious can mean real food with amazing flavor at a reasonable cost. This approach to eating is not about deprivation or starvation or boring, bland diet food. Rather, it is about amazing, delicious, fun, and easy-to-prepare food that makes you feel great.

We hope you will share these meals with your friends and family, and that they become your favorites for generations to come. By buying this book and putting your commitment to healthy eating into action, you too can become a part of the solution.

You now have all of the information you need to embark on your healthy eating journey. One last note: Let this cookbook bring out the inner culinary genius in you. While following recipes is often helpful and inspiring, you don't need recipes in order to eat well. I encourage you to start your own cooking revolution, whether you're following these recipes to a T, editing them to suit your own tastes (a little more garlic, a little less cumin), or abandoning them in favor of your own creations. Have fun, and happy eating!

7

The Basic Plan

BREAKFAST

STRAWBERRY-ALMOND-COCONUT SMOOTHIE

When selecting berries, especially strawberries, choose organic to prevent over-loading your system with toxic residue from fertilizers and pesticides. You can likely find frozen organic berries in your local supermarket year-round; they work great in your morning shake.

- 1 or 2 large ice cubes
- 2 tablespoons unsalted almond butter
- ¾ cup light unsweetened coconut milk
- ½ cup unsweetened almond milk
- ½ cup frozen organic strawberries
- 2 teaspoons chia seeds

Combine all of the ingredients in a blender and blend on high until smooth, 1 to 2 minutes. If the smoothie is too thick, add a little water and blend again until it reaches the desired consistency. Drink immediately.

Nutritional analysis per serving: Calories: 380, Fat: 29 g, Saturated Fat: 8 g, Cholesterol: 0 mg, Fiber: 9 g, Protein: 12 g, Carbohydrates: 13 g, Sodium: 150 mg

BLUEBERRY-NUT SMOOTHIE

Serves: 1

Prep Time:
5 minutes

Just 2 Brazil nuts will fulfill your daily need for selenium. Selenium is a power-ful antioxidant that helps your immune system stay resilient and also plays a role in a healthy functioning thyroid. Be sure to limit your intake of Brazil nuts to no more than 4 per day, as too much selenium can be bad for you.

- ½ cup frozen blueberries
- 2 raw Brazil nuts
- 4 raw walnuts
- 4 ounces non-GMO silken tofu
- 1 cup unsweetened hemp or almond milk
- ½ teaspoon fresh lemon juice
- ¼ teaspoon ground cinnamon
- pinch of sea salt
- 1 or 2 ice cubes

Combine all of the ingredients in a blender and blend on high until smooth, 1 to 2 minutes. If the smoothie is too thick, add a little water and blend again until it reaches the desired consistency. Drink immediately.

Nutritional analysis per serving: *Calories: 252, Fat: 21 g, Saturated Fat: 3 g, Cholesterol: 0 mg, Fiber: 5 g, Protein: 15 g, Carbohydrates: 18 g, Sodium: 248 mg*

Açai Smoothie

Serves: 1

Prep Time:
5 minutes

Açai is a type of palm tree native to the Amazon in Brazil. It boasts a load of antioxidants, amino acids, and omega fatty acids. It even contains protein! I love it because its nutrition profile helps put the brakes on the aging process by cooling inflammation and boosting metabolic function as well as eliminating harmful free radicals from our bodies.

- ¼ cup frozen blueberries
- ¼ cup frozen açai puree
- 1 (¼-inch) slice ginger, peeled
- 3 tablespoons unsweetened hemp protein powder
- 1 tablespoon coconut butter
- ½ cup full-fat unsweetened coconut milk
- 1 or 2 ice cubes (optional)

Combine all of the ingredients in a blender and blend on high speed until smooth, 1 to 2 minutes. If the smoothie is too thick, add a little water and blend again until it reaches the desired consistency. Drink immediately.

Nutritional analysis per serving: *Calories: 295 Fat: 21 g, Saturated Fat: 13 g, Cholesterol: 0 mg, Fiber: 8 g, Protein: 14 g, Carbohydrates: 16 g, Sodium: 250 mg*

CREAMY BERRY SMOOTHIE

Serves: 1

Prep Time:
5 minutes

I like plant-based protein such as hemp protein powder in my morning smoothie. It is hypoallergenic, which means most people will not have a low-grade inflammatory response to it as some do with soy or dairy. Hemp contains healthy omega fatty acids, protein, antioxidants, fiber, and minerals that support a healthy metabolism and energize your body for a productive morning.

- ¼ cup frozen organic strawberries
- ¼ cup frozen raspberries
- 4 ounces non-GMO silken tofu
- 2 tablespoon unsweetened hemp protein powder
- 1 teaspoon fresh lime juice
- 1 or 2 ice cubes (optional)

Combine all of the ingredients in a blender and blend on high speed until smooth, 1 to 2 minutes. If the smoothie is too thick, add a little water and blend again until it reaches the desired consistency. Drink immediately.

Nutritional analysis per serving: *Calories: 257, Fat: 6 g, Saturated Fat: 0 g, Cholesterol: 0 mg, Fiber: 9 g, Protein: 21 g, Carbohydrates: 31 g, Sodium: 13 mg*

Almond-Berry Smoothie

Serves: 1

Prep Time:
5 minutes

I love this recipe for those mornings when I feel like something refreshing and light yet need real-food energy to carry me through the day. The fiber, protein, and healthy fat in this smoothie keep me going until lunch.

- ¼ cup frozen raspberries
- ¼ cup frozen blackberries
- 2 tablespoons unsweetened hemp protein powder
- 1 tablespoon flaxseed
- 1 tablespoon unsalted almond butter
- ½ cup unsweetened almond milk
- 1 teaspoon fresh lemon juice
- 1 or 2 ice cubes (optional)

Combine all of the ingredients in a blender and blend on high speed until smooth, 1 to 2 minutes. If the smoothie is too thick, add a little water and blend again until it reaches the desired consistency. Drink immediately.

Nutritional analysis per serving: Calories: 341, Fat: 19 g, Saturated Fat: 2 g, Cholesterol: 0 mg, Fiber: 11 g, Protein: 21 g, Carbohydrates: 21 g, Sodium: 135 mg

COCOA-ALMOND SMOOTHIE

When selecting cocoa products, try to find raw cacao powder in your local market or order online. Raw cacao is less processed than cocoa and yields higher amounts of minerals, vitamins, healthy fats, and fiber.

- 2 or 3 large ice cubes
- 1¼ cups unsweetened almond milk
- 2 tablespoons unsalted almond butter
- 1 tablespoon chia seeds
- 2 teaspoons unsweetened cocoa powder
- 1 tablespoon coconut oil

Combine all of the ingredients in a blender and blend on high speed until smooth, 1 to 2 minutes. If the smoothie is too thick, add a little water and blend again until it reaches the desired consistency. Drink immediately.

Nutritional analysis per serving: *Calories: 430, Fat: 39 g, Saturated Fat: 14 g, Cholesterol: 0 mg, Fiber: 9 g, Protein: 10 g, Carbohydrates: 14 g, Sodium: 300 mg*

CRUSTLESS ASPARAGUS QUICHE

Serves: 4

Prep Time:
15 minutes

Cook Time:
20 minutes

I love a good quiche to start off my weekend. Incorporating vegetables and herbs into an egg dish is a creative way to enjoy a savory meal that works for breakfast, lunch, or dinner.

- 1¾ teaspoons sea salt
- 8 asparagus spears, trimmed
- 10 large omega-3 eggs
- 2 shallots, finely chopped
- ¼ cup lightly packed coarsely chopped fresh dill
- 2 teaspoons grapeseed oil
- 1 avocado, pitted, peeled, and sliced, for garnish

Preheat the oven to 425°F.

Bring a 3-quart saucepan of water to a boil over high heat. Add 1 teaspoon of the sea salt.

Add the asparagus to the boiling water and cook until bright green and crisp-tender, 1 to 2 minutes. Transfer the asparagus to a colander and rinse with cold water until cool. Dry the asparagus thoroughly with paper towels. Set aside.

In a large bowl, whisk together the eggs, shallots, dill, and remaining ¾ teaspoon salt.

Place a 9½ by 2-inch deep nonstick quiche pan with a removable bottom on a rimmed baking sheet. Wrap the bottom of the pan tightly with aluminum foil. Using a pastry brush, lightly grease the pan with the grapeseed oil.

Spread the asparagus evenly in the bottom of the pan. Pour the egg mixture over the asparagus.

Place the baking sheet in the center of the oven and bake until the quiche is puffed and golden and a toothpick inserted in the center comes out clean, 15 to 17 minutes. Cool for 10 minutes before removing from the pan.

Serve, garnished with sliced avocado.

Nutritional analysis per serving: *Calories: 210, Fat: 14 g, Saturated Fat: 3.5 g, Cholesterol: 450 mg, Fiber: 1 g, Protein: 16 g, Carbohydrates: 6 g, Sodium: 421 mg*

VEGETABLE HASH WITH FRIED EGGS

Serves: 4

Prep Time:
10 minutes

Cook Time:
30 minutes

If you don't have time to make this in the morning, make the hash a few days ahead, store it in the refrigerator, and then reheat it in a sauté pan or cast-iron skillet.

- 2 tablespoons extra-virgin olive oil
- 1 medium yellow onion, diced
- 1 medium white or green cabbage, diced
- 1 organic red bell pepper, seeded and diced
- 1 organic green bell pepper, seeded and diced
- 8 asparagus spears, trimmed and cut into ¼-inch pieces
- 2 scallions, thinly sliced
- ½ teaspoon dried oregano
- ½ teaspoon dried thyme
- ½ teaspoon dried sage
- ¼ teaspoon sea salt
- pinch of freshly ground black pepper
- 8 large omega-3 eggs
- ½ ripe avocado, pitted, peeled, and sliced, for garnish
- chopped fresh basil or parsley, for garnish

Preheat the oven to 400°F.

Heat the oil in a large oven-safe sauté pan or cast-iron skillet over medium heat for 30 seconds. Add the onion and sauté, stirring occasionally, until lightly caramelized and golden, 5 to 7 minutes.

Add the cabbage and sauté until soft and golden, 7 to 8 minutes. Add the bell peppers and sauté until they begin to caramelize, about 5 minutes. Add the asparagus and scallions and cook for an additional 1 to 2 minutes, or just until the asparagus turns bright green.

Season the vegetables with the dried herbs, salt, and black pepper. Make four small wells in the surface of the hash, each about the size of a lemon, and carefully break two eggs into each well.

Place the pan in the oven and bake until the eggs are set, 5 to 7 minutes. (Alternatively, you can poach or fry the eggs, then serve them on individual plates of hash.)

Garnish each egg with avocado and fresh herbs and serve.

Nutritional analysis per serving: Calories: 280, Fat: 19 g, Saturated Fat: 4 g, Cholesterol: 360 mg, Fiber: 5 g, Protein: 15 g, Carbohydrates: 14 g, Sodium: 290 mg

SOUTHWESTERN VEGETABLE FRITTATA

Serves: 4

Prep Time:
10 minutes

Cook Time:
35 minutes

Frittatas are a great way to use up leftovers, and you can feel free to add other cooked vegetables than the ones mentioned here. Try chopped cooked broccoli, grilled zucchini and bell peppers, or sautéed spinach.

- 8 large omega-3 eggs
- ½ teaspoon mild chili powder
- 1 tablespoon minced fresh chives and/or basil
- sea salt and freshly ground black pepper
- 1 tablespoon extra-virgin olive oil
- ¼ red onion, thinly sliced
- ½ small head white cabbage, finely diced
- 1 garlic clove, minced
- 2 cups tightly packed stemmed and finely shredded kale or other leafy green
- 16 roasted grape tomatoes (see Note)
- 1 ripe avocado, pitted, peeled, and diced, for garnish
- salsa, for garnish (optional)

Preheat the oven to 375°F.

In a bowl, whisk together the eggs, chili powder, herbs, ½ teaspoon salt, and a pinch of black pepper.

Heat the olive oil in an 8-inch nonstick oven-safe skillet over medium heat until shimmering.

Add the red onion to the pan and sauté for 1 minute, then add the cabbage. Sauté the cabbage until it's wilted and beginning to brown, about 5 minutes. Add the garlic and kale to the pan and cook until the kale is wilted and very soft, about 5 minutes more. Season the vegetables with a pinch of salt.

Pour the egg mixture over the vegetables and scatter the roasted tomatoes over the eggs. Place the pan in the oven and bake until the eggs are fully set but the center is just barely soft, 18 to 22 minutes. Remove the frittata from the oven and allow it to rest for 5 minutes. Cut into 4 wedges and serve, garnished with avocado and salsa, if desired.

Note: To make the roasted grape tomatoes, preheat the oven to 400°F. Toss a pint of grape or cherry tomatoes with 1 tablespoon of extra-virgin olive oil and a pinch of salt, and spread them out on a rimmed baking sheet. Roast the tomatoes until they are shriveled and starting to brown, about 30 minutes. Let them cool for 5 minutes, then transfer them to an airtight container and store in the refrigerator for up to 5 days. They can be added to salads, stews, and sauces, or mashed up with basil as a delicious topping for grilled meats and fish.

Nutritional analysis per serving (does not include salsa): *Calories: 240, Fat: 16 g, Saturated Fat: 3.5 g, Cholesterol: 360 mg, Fiber: 4 g, Protein: 15 g, Carbohydrates: 11 g, Sodium: 450 mg*

Asparagus and Mushroom Frittata with Tomato Coulis

Serves: 4

Prep Time:
20 minutes

Cook Time:
20 minutes

Coulis is a French culinary term to describe a thick puree. Here, the tomato coulis balances the pungent flavor of the onion and the earthiness of the mushrooms. This frittata will make you feel as if you just enjoyed brunch at your local brasserie without even leaving home!

- 2 tomatoes, cored and quartered
- 2 oil-packed sun-dried tomatoes
- 1 small garlic clove
- 1 teaspoon sea salt
- ½ teaspoon freshly ground black pepper
- 3 tablespoons extra-virgin olive oil
- 1 large red onion, finely chopped
- 1 pound asparagus, trimmed and cut on the bias into 1-inch pieces
- 8 ounces cremini mushrooms, trimmed and thinly sliced
- 6 large omega-3 eggs

To make the tomato coulis, combine the fresh tomatoes, sun-dried tomatoes, garlic, and ¼ teaspoon each salt and black pepper in a blender or food processor. Puree until smooth. Set aside.

Heat 2 tablespoons of the oil in a 9-inch nonstick skillet over medium heat until shimmering. Add the onion, sprinkle with ¼ teaspoon salt, and cook, stirring occasionally, until just translucent, about 7 minutes.

Add the asparagus and mushrooms, sprinkle with another ¼ teaspoon salt, and cook, stirring occasionally, until the asparagus is crisp-tender and the juices released by the mushrooms evaporate, about 6 minutes.

Meanwhile, in a bowl, whisk the eggs with the remaining ¼ teaspoon each salt and black pepper. Add the asparagus mixture to the eggs and stir gently.

Heat the remaining 1 tablespoon oil in the same skillet over medium heat until shimmering. Pour the egg mixture into the skillet and fold gently, pulling the cooked edges in to evenly cook the eggs.

When the egg mixture starts to set, spread it out in an even layer, cover, and cook until fully set, about 3 minutes. Uncover and loosen the frittata before inverting or sliding onto a serving plate. Cut into wedges and serve with the tomato coulis spooned over the top.

Nutritional analysis per serving: Calories: 260, Fat: 18 g, Saturated Fat: 3.5 g, Cholesterol: 270 mg, Fiber: 4 g, Protein: 14 g, Carbohydrates: 15 g, Sodium: 523 mg

WILD MUSHROOM AND LEEK FRITTATA

Serves: 4

Prep Time:
15 minutes

Cook Time:
35 minutes

While it makes a great breakfast, a frittata can also be served with a green salad for lunch or even a light dinner. Make sure your wild mushrooms come from a reputable source—a farmers' market is best. Don't be intimidated by using leeks; they're simple to clean and delicious.

- 4 tablespoons plus 1 teaspoon grapeseed oil
- 1 large leek, cut into ½-inch-thick slices
- 6 ounces wild mushrooms, stemmed and cut into ¼-inch-thick slices
- 2 teaspoons fresh thyme
- ¾ teaspoon sea salt
- pinch of cayenne pepper, or to taste
- 8 large omega-3 eggs, beaten
- ½ small bunch chives, thinly sliced, for garnish

Preheat the oven to 425°F.

Heat 1 teaspoon of the oil in a large oven-safe skillet over medium-low heat until shimmering. Add the leek and cook until tender, 6 to 8 minutes. Transfer the leek to a bowl and set aside.

Add 2 tablespoons of the oil to the skillet and raise the temperature to medium-high. When the skillet is hot, add half of the mushrooms; cook, stirring occasionally, until they are deep golden-brown, 3 to 4 minutes. If the bottom of the pan begins to get dark, add ¼ cup water and use a flexible rubber spatula to loosen the dark bits. Add the cooked mushrooms to the reserved leeks.

Return the skillet to the heat. Repeat the process with the remaining 2 tablespoons oil and the remaining mushrooms. Once the second batch of mushrooms is cooked, return the leek and mushroom mixture to the skillet.

Add the thyme, salt, and cayenne pepper to the skillet and stir to combine.

Remove the skillet from the heat, add the eggs, and quickly stir to combine the ingredients.

Place the skillet in the oven on the center rack. Cook until golden brown, puffed, and set (a toothpick inserted in the center should come out clean), 13 to 15 minutes. Allow to cool for 5 minutes before running a flexible rubber spatula around the edges and then carefully underneath the frittata to loosen it from the bottom of the pan. Slide the frittata onto a plate, cut into wedges, and serve garnished with about 1 tablespoon of chives per wedge.

Note: The frittata can be served cold. Allow it to come to room temperature before covering and chilling.

Nutritional analysis per serving: *Calories: 300, Fat: 24 g, Saturated Fat: 4 g, Cholesterol: 360 mg, Fiber: 2 g, Protein: 13 g, Carbohydrates: 8 g, Sodium: 550 mg*

Turkey Sausage Patties

Serves: 4

Prep Time:
10 minutes

Cook Time:
10 minutes

Enjoy a serving of sausage patties with a fried egg or scrambled eggs mixed with chopped cooked asparagus and some fresh berries alongside.

- 1 pound lean ground turkey
- 2½ teaspoons fennel seeds
- 1 teaspoon dried oregano
- 1 teaspoon dried thyme
- 1 teaspoon sweet paprika
- ½ teaspoon crushed red pepper flakes
- ½ teaspoon sea salt
- ¼ teaspoon freshly ground black pepper
- 1 tablespoon avocado or grapeseed oil
- 2 cups fresh berries

In a bowl, combine the ground turkey and all of the spices, salt, and black pepper. Use your hands to combine the mixture, making sure the spices are well mixed into the ground turkey. Form the meat into 8 equal-size patties.

Heat the oil in a large nonstick skillet over medium-high heat until shimmering. Sauté the patties until brown on both sides and cooked through, 8 to 10 minutes, using a heat-safe spatula to press down and flatten the patties a few times as they cook. Check to make sure the turkey is fully cooked by cutting into the center of one patty (no pink should remain) or checking that the internal temperature measures 165°F.

Serve 2 patties with ½ cup berries.

Nutritional analysis per serving: *Calories: 252, Fat: 13 g, Saturated Fat: 3 g, Cholesterol: 84 mg, Fiber: 3 g, Protein: 22 g, Carbohydrates: 12 g, Sodium: 321 mg*

POACHED EGGS OVER SPINACH WITH BRAISED ARTICHOKE BOTTOMS

Serves: 4

Prep Time:
15 minutes

Cook Time:
15 minutes

Poaching is a fast and healthy way to cook eggs. Because the yolk is not exposed to high heat for too long, the essential fats as well as important fat-soluble vitamins and antioxidants—like lutein—do not break down.

- 2 teaspoons extra-virgin olive oil
- 10 cups loosely packed stemmed organic spinach
- sea salt
- 2 (13.5-ounce) cans artichoke bottoms, rinsed and drained
- 8 large omega-3 eggs, plus 1 yolk
- ½ cup Mayonnaise (page 299) or Vegenaise
- 1 teaspoon Dijon mustard
- grated zest and juice of 1 lemon
- 1 garlic clove, halved
- ⅛ teaspoon cayenne pepper
- 2 teaspoons white vinegar or additional fresh lemon juice, for poaching
- paprika, for garnish

Preheat the broiler. Line a baking sheet with aluminum foil and brush the foil with 1 teaspoon of the oil. Set aside.

In a large nonstick skillet, heat the remaining 1 teaspoon oil over medium-high heat until shimmering. Add the spinach and toss until slightly wilted. Season with a pinch of salt. Cover and cook for 1 minute. Transfer to a colander and press out any excess liquid from the greens.

Slice off the underside of each artichoke bottom so that they sit flat. Place the artichoke bottoms on the prepared baking sheet and broil until warm and slightly golden, about 3 minutes. Set aside.

While the artichokes cook, combine the egg yolk, mayonnaise, mustard, lemon zest and juice, garlic, cayenne, ½ teaspoon salt, and 2 tablespoons cold water in a food processor and pulse until the mixture reaches a creamy, sauce-like consistency.

Bring 4 cups of water to a simmer in a medium saucepan over medium-high heat. Add the white vinegar to the simmering water. Crack 1 egg into a small bowl and gently tip the egg into the water. Quickly repeat with 3 more eggs, being careful not to let the eggs touch. Cook until the whites are set and the yolks are runny, 2 to 3 minutes. With a slotted spoon, transfer the eggs to a plate lined with paper towels to drain. Repeat with the remaining 4 eggs.

Place two artichoke bottoms on each plate. Top each with cooked spinach and an egg, then a spoonful of sauce. Garnish with a sprinkle of paprika and serve.

Nutritional analysis per serving: *Calories: 342, Fat: 28 g, Saturated Fat: 6 g, Cholesterol: 432 mg, Fiber: 13 g, Protein: 19 g, Carbohydrates: 20 g, Sodium: 580 mg*

SPINACH-MUSHROOM-ASPARAGUS STRATA

Serves: 4

Prep Time:
15 minutes

Cook Time:
1 hour

Concerned about eggs raising your cholesterol? Don't be! This nutrition myth constantly surprises my patients. It turns out that cholesterol from food is not the culprit—sugar is! By enjoying seven to eight omega-3 eggs per week, you increase your antioxidant intake and receive healthy amounts of fat, protein, and nutrition—all of which help lower your cholesterol, not raise it.

- 3 teaspoons coconut oil
- 2 pounds cremini mushrooms, trimmed and sliced
- 2 (5-ounce) bags organic baby spinach
- 2 garlic cloves, minced
- 1½ tablespoons pine nuts
- 1 pound asparagus, trimmed
- 8 large omega-3 eggs
- ⅓ cup unsweetened almond milk
- 2 tablespoons nutritional yeast, plus more for optional garnish
- 1 scallion, finely chopped
- 1 jalapeño, seeded and finely chopped (optional)
- ¼ teaspoon sea salt
- ¼ teaspoon freshly ground black pepper

Preheat the oven to 350°F. Lightly coat an 8-inch square baking dish with 1 teaspoon of the coconut oil; set aside.

Warm 1 teaspoon of the coconut oil in a large nonstick sauté pan over medium-high heat until shimmering. Add the mushrooms and sauté until they have released their liquid and that liquid has evaporated, 8 to 10 minutes. Transfer the mushrooms to a bowl and set aside.

In the same pan, warm the remaining 1 teaspoon coconut oil over medium heat until shimmering. Add half of the spinach, stirring constantly until wilted, 2 to 3 minutes. Add the remaining spinach, stirring again and cooking until wilted, another 2 minutes. Stir in the garlic and pine nuts; cook for 30 seconds. Remove the pan from the heat and set aside.

Transfer half of the mushrooms to the bottom of the prepared baking dish. Top with half of the spinach. Layer half of the asparagus spears on top of the spinach. Repeat with the remaining mushrooms, spinach, and asparagus.

In a small bowl, whisk together the eggs and almond milk. Add the nutritional yeast, scallion, jalapeño (if using), salt, and black pepper, whisking to combine. Pour the egg mixture evenly into the baking dish.

Bake until the center is firm to the touch, 40 to 50 minutes. A little of the moisture from the vegetables will rise to the top; blot with a paper towel, if desired.

Cut the strata into 4 squares and serve, garnished with additional nutritional yeast, if desired.

Nutritional analysis per serving: *Calories: 293, Fat: 15 g, Saturated Fat: 5 g, Cholesterol: 350 mg, Fiber: 9 g, Protein: 25 g, Carbohydrates: 25 g, Sodium: 318 mg*

SPICY SCRAMBLED TOFU WITH ZUCCHINI AND CILANTRO

Serves: 4

Prep Time:
10 minutes

Cook Time:
20 minutes

I encourage my community to avoid all genetically modified soy because of the hazardous health effects it carries. Most GMO soy cultivated in this country is made to resist a chemical pesticide called glyphosate, which ultimately leaves a residue on the soy we consume. Avoid this potentially harmful chemical and other toxins by choosing only GMO-free soy foods.

- 5 tablespoons extra-virgin olive oil
- 3 small zucchini, cut into 1-inch cubes
- 1 small yellow onion, chopped
- 3 garlic cloves, minced
- 1 green Thai chile, seeded and minced
- 1 teaspoon grated fresh ginger
- ¼ teaspoon crushed red pepper flakes
- 1 pound organic spinach, stemmed
- 1 (14-ounce) package non-GMO extra-firm tofu, drained and crumbled
- ½ teaspoon sea salt
- ¼ cup roughly chopped fresh cilantro

Heat 3 tablespoons of the oil in a 12-inch skillet over high heat until shimmering. Add the zucchini and cook until browned on all sides and tender, 6 to 8 minutes. Transfer to a large bowl.

Add the onion, garlic, chile, ginger, and pepper flakes to the skillet and cook until the onion is translucent, 3 to 5 minutes. Add the onion mixture to the bowl with the zucchini.

Add the spinach to the skillet and cook, stirring often, until just wilted, 2 to 3 minutes. Add the spinach to the zucchini and onion mixture.

Heat the remaining 2 tablespoons oil in the skillet over medium heat until shimmering. Add the tofu and cook, stirring, until heated through, 3 to 5 minutes. Add the tofu to the zucchini mixture. Season with the salt, stir in the chopped cilantro, and serve.

Nutritional analysis per serving: *Calories: 320, Fat: 23 g, Saturated Fat: 3.5 g, Cholesterol: 0 mg, Fiber: 8 g, Protein: 14 g, Carbohydrates: 20 g, Sodium: 340 mg*

LUNCH

Dr. Hyman's Super Salad Bar

Why go to a salad bar when you can create your own at home? As always, preparation is the key to a successful detox. To get our kitchens and ourselves prepared to enjoy a delicious salad from home, be sure to take a little time to set up your own salad bar fixings. Here's what to do:

■ Wash and cut veggies into convenient salad-size bits and store them in sealed glass containers all in one location in your refrigerator. Cut enough for 2 to 3 days and repeat throughout the 10 days as needed for freshness. Add different veggies at least twice a week for variety.

■ Make a salad for lunch the night before so you can grab-and-go on your way out the door. Store dressing in a separate container.

■ Store items not requiring refrigeration in small glass jars, preferably on a single shelf so they're easy to find. Toasted and raw nuts and seeds stay fresh for weeks at room temperature when sealed in glass jars.

■ Ready, set, prep: Pick a variety of items from the list below and add them to your shopping list each week. Start by choosing your greens. Consider mixing various types of greens—I like having some romaine with arugula to balance out texture. (Skip iceberg lettuce; it is hardly green and has almost no nutrients.) Then choose your veggies, protein, healthy fats, and dressing. Select different options each day to keep your palate happy.

GREENS (2 CUPS PER SALAD)
■ Arugula
■ Spinach (organic when possible)
■ Romaine
■ Watercress

- Kale
- Mixed baby greens

VEGETABLES (1 TO 2 CUPS PER SALAD EXCEPT AS NOTED)

- Cucumbers (organic when possible)
- Bell peppers: red, green, yellow (organic when possible)
- Sprouts: sunflower, pea shoots, clover, etc.
- Tomatoes: grape, cherry (organic when possible)
- Carrots
- Broccoli
- Cauliflower
- Cabbage: red, napa, etc.
- Mushrooms
- Snap peas (organic when possible)
- Steamed asparagus
- Artichoke hearts (packed in water in glass jars)
- Hearts of palm (packed in water in glass jars)
- Zucchini
- Roasted eggplant
- Roasted or steamed beets (¼ to ½ cup)
- Red onions (¼ to ½ cup)
- Scallions (¼ to ½ cup)
- Herbs: parsley, basil, oregano, dill, cilantro, mint, oregano, etc. (¼ cup fresh and/or 1 teaspoon dried)

PROTEIN (4 TO 6 OUNCES)

- Canned fish (in water): salmon, sardines, herring, etc. (Skip tuna; it has too much mercury.)
- Chicken (baked or roasted)
- Turkey (baked or roasted)
- Tofu
- Tempeh
- Hard-boiled eggs (2)
- Cooked shrimp or other seafood

HEALTHY FATS (CHOOSE ONE)

- Avocado (¼ to ½)
- Nuts, raw: almonds, cashews, walnuts, hazelnuts, pecans, etc. (¼ cup)
- Seeds, raw: flax, chia, hemp, sunflower, pumpkin, sesame, etc. (¼ cup)
- Kalamata olives (¼ cup)

DRESSING (1 TO 2 TABLESPOONS PER SALAD)

Start by mixing oil (extra-virgin olive oil, flaxseed oil, walnut oil, or avocado oil) and fresh lemon or lime juice or vinegar (or a combination) at a ratio of two-thirds oil to one-third lemon or vinegar. Whisk in any of these to taste:

- Dijon mustard
- Seasonings, including salt and black pepper; fresh or dried herbs such as basil, oregano, or rosemary; and minced garlic or onion. For creamy dressing, add avocado or tahini (sesame paste).

BLANCHED ASPARAGUS WITH SOFT-BOILED EGGS

Serves: 4

Prep Time:
5 minutes

Cook Time:
10 minutes

I love anchovies. Contrary to popular belief they don't taste "fishy" but rather slightly savory and salty. A little anchovy packs a lot of flavor, so you don't need many to get a burst of flavor from these heart-healthy fish.

- 8 large omega-3 eggs
- sea salt
- 2 pounds asparagus, trimmed
- ¼ cup halved Niçoise olives
- 4 oil-packed anchovy fillets, coarsely chopped
- 2 tablespoons extra-virgin olive oil
- ¼ cup roughly chopped fresh basil
- ¼ teaspoon freshly ground black pepper

Put the eggs in a large saucepan and add enough cold water to cover by 1 inch. Bring the water to a boil over medium heat; remove from the heat and cover. Let stand for 2 minutes (see Note). Use a slotted spoon to transfer the eggs to a bowl; reserve the hot water in the pan. Cover the eggs with cold water and set aside.

Return the water in the pan to a boil over medium-high heat and add 2 teaspoons salt. Add the asparagus and cook until bright green and almost crisp-tender, about 4 minutes. Drain and arrange in a single layer on four serving plates. Scatter the olives and anchovies evenly over the asparagus.

Lightly crack 2 eggs over each bed of asparagus and scoop them out, letting the yolks run over the asparagus. Sprinkle the eggs with a pinch of salt. Drizzle the olive oil over each serving and scatter the basil leaves on top. Sprinkle with the black pepper and serve.

Note: If you prefer a firmer egg, leave the eggs in the hot water for 3 minutes for medium-boiled and 8 minutes for hard-boiled.

Nutritional analysis per serving: *Calories: 281, Fat: 19 g, Saturated Fat: 4 g, Cholesterol: 363 mg, Fiber: 5 g, Protein: 18 g, Carbohydrates: 12 g, Sodium: 507 mg*

CHERRY TOMATO AND TOFU SALAD

Serves: 4

Prep Time: 10 minutes, plus resting time

This salad gets better the longer it sits, as the tofu soaks up the dressing and tomato juices. It is lovely served on a bed of peppery arugula leaves.

- 2 teaspoons gluten-free, low-sodium tamari
- 2 teaspoons toasted sesame oil
- 1 teaspoon balsamic vinegar
- 2 tablespoons extra-virgin olive oil
- 3 pints cherry or grape tomatoes, halved
- 3 tablespoons raw pumpkin seeds
- 2 teaspoons sesame seeds
- 1 (14-ounce) package non-GMO extra-firm tofu, drained and cut into 1-inch cubes
- ¼ teaspoon sea salt
- ¼ teaspoon freshly ground black pepper
- 1 avocado, pitted, peeled, and chopped
- ¼ cup julienned fresh mint

In a large bowl, combine the tamari, sesame oil, and balsamic vinegar. Whisk in the olive oil.

Add the tomatoes to the bowl, stirring to combine with the dressing. Stir in the pumpkin and sesame seeds.

Add the tofu cubes and season with the salt and black pepper. Gently toss. Let sit for 30 minutes at room temperature, so the tofu absorbs the dressing. (The salad can also sit in the refrigerator, covered, for up to 1 day prior to serving.)

Top with the chopped avocado and mint and serve.

Nutritional analysis per serving: *Calories: 350, Fat: 26 g, Saturated Fat: 3.5 g, Cholesterol: 0 mg, Fiber: 7 g, Protein: 15 g, Carbohydrates: 17 g, Sodium: 310 mg*

Serves: 4

Prep Time:
15 minutes,
plus resting
time

THAI TOFU AND AVOCADO SALAD WITH CHILE-LIME DRESSING

Look for organic, extra-firm tofu, which has a pleasing chewy texture and will also soak up the dressing really well.

- 1 (14-ounce) package non-GMO extra-firm tofu, drained and cut into ½-inch cubes
- ¼ teaspoon ground turmeric
- 2 tablespoons extra-virgin olive oil
- 1 tablespoon fresh lime juice
- 1 tablespoon Thai fish sauce
- Pinch red pepper flakes
- 2 cups shredded napa or green cabbage
- 1 cup thinly sliced cucumber
- 4 plum tomatoes, cut into eighths
- ¼ cup thinly sliced red onion or shallot
- ½ cup roughly chopped mixed fresh herbs (such as cilantro, mint, and/or basil)
- 2 tablespoons slivered or sliced almonds
- ½ avocado, pitted, peeled, and diced

Place the tofu in a large salad bowl and sprinkle with the turmeric. Toss well to combine. Set aside.

In a small bowl, whisk together the olive oil, lime juice, fish sauce, and red pepper flakes. Pour half of the dressing over the tofu and set aside for 30 minutes to allow it to marinate while you cut up the vegetables. Set aside the remaining dressing.

Add the cabbage, cucumber, tomatoes, and onion to the tofu. Add the remaining dressing to the salad and toss well to combine. Garnish with the herbs, almonds, and avocado and serve.

Nutritional analysis per serving: *Calories: 240, Fat: 17 g, Saturated Fat: 3 g, Cholesterol: 0 mg, Fiber: 5 g, Protein: 13 g, Carbohydrates: 11 g, Sodium: 370 mg*

BRUSSELS SPROUTS AND BROCCOLI SLAW WITH SEARED SCALLOPS

Serves: 4

Prep Time:
15 minutes

Cook Time:
10 minutes

Ounce for ounce, broccoli stems have the same nutrition as the florets. When you eat real food you can be sure that for the most part, the whole food can be consumed and will provide nutrition that our bodies can use to flourish.

- 1 pound Brussels sprouts, trimmed
- 1¾ pounds broccoli, stems peeled, florets cut into bite-size pieces
- ¼ cup julienned fresh basil
- ¼ cup fresh lemon juice
- 4 tablespoons balsamic vinegar
- 3 tablespoons extra-virgin olive oil
- sea salt and freshly ground black pepper
- 16 large sea scallops, patted dry, tough muscles discarded

Fit the shredding blade into a food processor. Process the Brussels sprouts and broccoli stems until finely shredded. Transfer to a large bowl. Add the basil, lemon juice, 2 tablespoons of the vinegar, 1 tablespoon of the oil, ¼ teaspoon salt, and a pinch of black pepper. Toss until mixed well. Set the slaw aside.

Heat 1 tablespoon of the oil in a large skillet over high heat until shimmering. Season the scallops with ¼ teaspoon salt and ½ teaspoon black pepper. Add the scallops to the skillet in a single layer without crowding; work in batches, if necessary. Cook until dark brown on the bottom, 1 to 2 minutes, and then flip and brown the other side, 1 to 2 minutes more. Transfer to a plate.

Add the remaining 1 tablespoon oil to the skillet and heat until shimmering. Add the broccoli florets in an even layer. Sprinkle with a pinch each of salt and black pepper. Add 2 tablespoons of water, cover, and cook until the broccoli is crisp-tender and browned on the bottom, about 3 minutes. Transfer to the slaw.

Add the remaining 2 tablespoons vinegar to the skillet and simmer until slightly thickened, about 30 seconds. To serve, divide the slaw among four serving plates, top with 4 scallops per plate, and drizzle with the reduced balsamic.

Nutritional analysis per serving: *Calories: 325, Fat: 13 g, Saturated Fat: 2 g, Cholesterol: 37 mg, Fiber: 10 g, Protein: 29 g, Carbohydrates: 30 g, Sodium: 570 mg*

FENNEL SALAD WITH ROAST COD FILLETS

Serves: 4

Prep Time:
10 minutes

Cook Time:
30 minutes

Cod is one of my favorite fish because it is mild yet firm and flaky, so it can take on the flavors of your meal, making for a great canvas. Enjoy the health benefits of cod in this easy-to-make, delicious salad.

- 2 fennel bulbs, trimmed and julienned
- 4 tablespoons plus 1 teaspoon grapeseed oil
- sea salt and freshly ground black pepper
- 2 bell peppers (red and/or yellow), seeded and julienned
- 1 large yellow onion, cut into 8 wedges
- 2 tablespoons sweet paprika
- 2 (12-ounce) wild-caught cod fillets
- 1 tablespoons extra-virgin olive oil
- 1 tablespoon balsamic vinegar
- 1 teaspoon Dijon mustard
- 2 small heads Boston lettuce, roughly torn

Preheat the oven to 450°F. Line two rimmed baking sheets with aluminum foil.

In a medium bowl, toss the fennel with 2 tablespoons of the grapeseed oil, ½ teaspoon salt, and a pinch of black pepper. Spread evenly on one of the lined baking sheets.

Put the bell peppers and onions in the same bowl and toss with another 2 tablespoons grapeseed oil, ½ teaspoon salt, and a pinch of black pepper. Spread evenly on the other lined baking sheet.

Roast the fennel on the bottom rack of the oven and the bell peppers and onions on the middle rack until the fennel has browned on the bottom, 12 to 15 minutes. Give all of the vegetables a toss to prevent burning and continue to cook until they are all golden brown, another 5 to 7 minutes. Remove from the oven, transfer to a large bowl, and set aside.

In a small bowl, whisk the paprika into ¼ cup cold water.

Remove the foil and brush one of the baking sheets with the remaining 1 teaspoon grapeseed oil and place the cod fillets on the sheet. Baste with about half of the paprika mixture. Roast until the cod is opaque throughout, basting again with the remaining paprika mixture halfway through. Fish typically takes about 12 minutes to cook per inch of thickness.

While the fish is baking, whisk together the olive oil, vinegar, mustard, and a pinch of salt in a small bowl. Add to the bowl of roasted vegetables and toss to coat.

Divide the lettuce among four serving plates and top with the roasted vegetables.

When the fish is done, use a fork to gently flake the fillets into bite-size pieces. Arrange the cod on top of the fennel salad and serve.

Nutritional analysis per serving: *Calories: 410, Fat: 21 g, Saturated Fat: 2.5 g, Cholesterol: 75 mg, Fiber: 9 g, Protein: 30 g, Carbohydrates: 23 g, Sodium: 490 mg*

GREEK SALAD WITH SPANISH MACKEREL

This salad is made for your 10-Day Detox Diet because it contains ingredients that are powerful detoxification agents. Onion, oregano, lemon, mackerel, olive oil, and vegetables contain potent nutrients to boost your metabolism.

- 1 tablespoon minced fresh oregano
- ¼ cup extra-virgin olive oil
- 4 (6-ounce) boneless wild Spanish mackerel fillets
- sea salt and freshly ground black pepper
- 2 large heads romaine lettuce, chopped
- ¾ cup diced heirloom tomatoes
- 1 cucumber, diced
- 1 large yellow bell pepper, seeded and very thinly sliced
- ¼ red onion, very thinly sliced
- ½ cup pitted Kalamata olives
- ¼ cup fresh lemon juice

Heat a well-seasoned stovetop grill pan over medium heat.

In a large bowl, whisk the chopped oregano into the oil.

Rub 1 tablespoon of the oregano-oil mixture all over the mackerel fillets. Season the fillets with ½ teaspoon salt and ¼ teaspoon black pepper. Place the fillets on the hot grill pan and grill until the flesh is just opaque throughout, about 5 minutes, turning once during grilling. Transfer to a cutting board and cut each fillet into thirds.

Add the lettuce, tomatoes, cucumber, bell pepper, onion, and olives to the remaining oregano-oil mixture. Sprinkle with a pinch each of salt and black pepper. Toss until well coated. Add the lemon juice and toss again. Divide the salad among four serving plates, top with the grilled mackerel, and serve.

Nutritional analysis per serving: *Calories: 460, Fat: 29 g, Saturated Fat: 5 g, Cholesterol: 130 mg, Fiber: 4 g, Protein: 36 g, Carbohydrates: 15 g, Sodium: 550 mg*

MUSTARD GREENS WITH GRILLED SALMON

Serves: 4

Prep Time:
25 minutes

Cook Time:
10 minutes

I love any recipe that has lemon or lime juice for the flavor-enhancing effects it has on the entire meal, so the fact that this recipe has both makes it a favorite in my home. If you prefer, feel free to substitute any hearty greens for the mustard greens, such as kale or turnip greens.

- juice of 1 lemon, plus grated zest of ½ lemon
- juice of 2 limes, plus grated zest of 1 lime
- 2½ tablespoons extra-virgin olive oil
- sea salt and freshly ground black pepper
- 1 to 2 large bunches mustard greens, roughly torn
- ½ cup parsley leaves
- ¼ small red onion, thinly sliced
- coconut oil, for coating grill
- 1 tablespoon Dijon mustard
- 4 (4- to 6-ounce) boneless, skin-on wild salmon fillets

In a small bowl, whisk together the citrus juices and zests.

In a separate small bowl prepare the dressing by whisking together 2 tablespoons of the citrus mixture, the olive oil, ¼ teaspoon salt, and a pinch of black pepper.

Place the greens in a large bowl, add the dressing, and gently massage the greens with your hands until the salad has wilted to almost half its original size, 2 to 3 minutes. Stir in the parsley and onion and set aside.

Prepare the grill for medium to medium-high heat, or heat a well-seasoned stovetop grill pan over medium-high heat. Lightly coat the grill or grill pan with coconut oil to prevent sticking.

In a small bowl, whisk together the mustard, remaining citrus mixture, and ¼ teaspoon each salt and black pepper. Using a spoon or a brush, spread the mustard mixture over the flesh side of the salmon fillets. Place the salmon fillets, skin-side up, on the grill or grill pan. Cook to the desired doneness, 4 to 5 minutes per side.

Divide the salad among four serving plates, place a fillet on each plate, and serve.

Nutritional analysis per serving: *Calories: 290, Fat: 16 g, Saturated Fat: 2 g, Cholesterol: 60 mg, Fiber: 6 g, Protein: 27 g, Carbohydrates: 11 g, Sodium: 480 mg*

SHRIMP AND SNOW PEA SALAD

Serves: 4

Prep Time:
30 minutes,
plus marinating
time

Cook Time:
5 minutes

This salad celebrates one of my favorite low-glycemic vegetables—jicama. Jicama (pronounced hee-ka-ma) is a nutrition powerhouse of fiber, potassium, vitamin C, and other antioxidants. It also contains the fiber inulin, which is a prebiotic that helps nourish our intestinal tract, allowing for healthy gut flora to flourish. A healthy microbiome is important for immunity, disease prevention, mood, and even keeping cravings away.

- ½ teaspoon sea salt
- 1 pound snow peas, trimmed and julienned
- 1 pound medium shrimp, peeled and deveined
- 2 teaspoons grated fresh lime zest
- 1 cup fresh lime juice (from 8 to 10 limes)
- ¼ cup extra-virgin olive oil
- 1 or 2 red chiles (such as Anaheim or Fresno), seeded and minced
- 1 small shallot, thinly sliced
- ½ cup chopped jicama
- ⅓ cup chopped fresh cilantro

Bring a 5-quart pot of water to a boil over high heat. Add ¼ teaspoon of the salt.

Add the peas to the boiling water and cook until bright green yet still crisp, about 1 minute. Remove the peas from the boiling water using a strainer, transfer to a colander, and immediately rinse with cold water until cooled. Keep the water boiling.

Line a rimmed baking sheet with paper towels and spread the peas onto the baking sheet. Pat dry and set aside.

Set up an ice bath by placing about 6 cups of ice and 2 cups of cold water in a large bowl.

Add the shrimp to the boiling water. Cover the pot, turn off the heat, and let the shrimp cook for 1 minute or until they are opaque and slightly pink.

Using a slotted spoon, transfer the shrimp to the ice bath and let sit 5 minutes to cool. Cut the shrimp in half lengthwise.

Combine the lime zest, juice, oil, chiles, shallot, and remaining ¼ teaspoon salt in a large bowl and stir. Add the cooled shrimp to the lime juice mixture, toss to combine, cover, and refrigerate for at least 30 minutes to marinate.

When ready to serve, add the snow peas, jicama, and cilantro to the shrimp mixture, and toss to combine. Divide among four serving plates and serve immediately.

Nutritional analysis per serving: *Calories: 330, Fat: 16 g, Saturated Fat: 2 g, Cholesterol: 215 mg, Fiber: 4 g, Protein: 27 g, Carbohydrates: 20 g, Sodium: 660 mg*

Niçoise Salad with Poached Salmon

Serves: 4

Prep Time:
25 minutes

Cook Time:
20 minutes

There is nothing I enjoy more than sharing a meal with friends and family, especially on the weekend. Sunday brunch is a great time to connect with the people you love, and this salad is easy to make, satisfying, and delicious for those special moments.

- 4 large omega-3 eggs
- 1 (9-ounce) package frozen artichoke hearts, thawed
- 8 ounces haricots verts, trimmed
- 1 lemon, thinly sliced
- 3 to 4 parsley sprigs
- 4 (4- to 6-ounce) boneless, skin-on wild salmon fillets
- sea salt and freshly ground black pepper
- 5 oil-packed anchovy fillets
- 2 tablespoons anchovy oil or extra-virgin olive oil
- 1½ tablespoons cider vinegar
- 8 to 10 Bibb lettuce leaves
- 1 pint cherry or grape tomatoes, halved
- ¼ cup Kalamata olives, pitted

Put the eggs in a large saucepan and add enough cold water to cover by 1 inch. Bring the water to a boil over medium heat, remove from the heat, and cover. Let stand for 12 minutes. Transfer the eggs to a bowl using a slotted spoon and cover with cold water. When the eggs have cooled, peel them and cut them into halves. Set aside.

Bring the water back to a boil over medium heat. Add the artichoke hearts and cook until tender, about 5 minutes. Using a slotted spoon, transfer the artichoke hearts to a small bowl. Add the haricots verts to the boiling water and cook until tender, 2 to 3 minutes. Prepare a water bath while the beans cook by filling a bowl with half ice cubes and half cold water. Drain the beans and add them to the water bath.

Pour 1 inch of water into a large skillet, along with the lemon slices and parsley. Bring the water to a boil over high heat. Season the salmon fillets with a pinch of salt and gently add them, skin-side down, to the water. Cover, reduce the heat to medium, and cook to the desired doneness, about 8 minutes. Carefully remove the salmon from the water and set aside.

Finely dice one of the anchovies and place in a small bowl. Add the oil, vinegar, ¼ teaspoon salt, and ½ teaspoon black pepper and whisk to combine all of the ingredients.

Line a large platter with lettuce leaves and top with the artichoke hearts, haricots verts, eggs, tomatoes, olives, and the remaining 4 anchovy fillets. Pour the dressing over the vegetables on the platter. Place the poached salmon on top of the salad and serve.

Nutritional analysis per serving: *Calories: 251, Fat: 17 g, Saturated Fat: 3 g, Cholesterol: 228 mg, Fiber: 7 g, Protein: 12 g, Carbohydrates: 16 g, Sodium: 564 mg*

Salmon Salad Wraps

Serves: 4

Prep Time:
20 minutes

Cook Time:
5 minutes

When you trade a less nutritious food for a higher-quality food without losing the personality of the dish, I call it a "swap." In this recipe, swap that blood sugar–spiking flour tortilla for crisp butter lettuce to enjoy a low-glycemic meal that satisfies both your taste buds and your waistline.

- 1 teaspoon sea salt
- juice of 1 lemon
- 2 (8-ounce) boneless, skinless wild salmon fillets
- 1 large yellow bell pepper, seeded and finely chopped
- 2 tablespoons finely chopped red onion
- 1 tablespoon finely chopped jalapeño
- 1 tablespoon rinsed capers, finely chopped
- 3 tablespoons fresh lime juice
- 1 tablespoon extra-virgin olive oil
- 2 tablespoons finely chopped fresh cilantro
- 12 butter lettuce leaves
- 2 avocados, pitted, peeled, and sliced

In a large skillet, bring 6 cups of water and ½ teaspoon of the salt to a boil over high heat. Add the lemon juice. Gently slide the salmon fillets into the boiling water. Reduce to a low simmer and poach until the salmon is cooked through and opaque, about 5 minutes. Remove from the water and set aside to cool to room temperature, 5 to 10 minutes. When cooled, flake into small pieces.

Meanwhile, in a large bowl, combine the bell pepper, onion, jalapeño, capers, lime juice, oil, and remaining ½ teaspoon salt and mix well. Let the salad stand while the salmon cooks and cools. Then gently fold the salmon and cilantro into the salad.

Divide the lettuce leaves among four serving plates. Then divide the salmon mixture into 12 portions and spoon a portion onto each leaf. Top the salmon mixture with the sliced avocado, fold the lettuce around the salmon and avocado to form a wrap, and then serve seam-side down.

Nutritional analysis per serving: *Calories: 370, Fat: 26 g, Saturated Fat: 4 g, Cholesterol: 60 mg, Fiber: 8 g, Protein: 25 g, Carbohydrates: 14 g, Sodium: 550 mg*

SEAWEED SALAD WITH POACHED SHRIMP

Serves: 4

Prep Time:
10 minutes

Cook Time:
3 minutes

You can substitute 1 pound of squid for the shrimp. Buy it cleaned, then cut the bodies into ¼-inch-thick rings and the tentacles in half lengthwise. Cook just until the tentacles curl and stiffen, about 30 seconds. Drain and immediately rinse under cold water until cool.

- 1 cup shredded dried wakame seaweed
- 1 cup shredded dried kombu seaweed
- 1 pound large shrimp, peeled and deveined
- 3 tablespoons gluten-free, low-sodium tamari
- 2 tablespoons apple cider vinegar
- 1 tablespoon toasted sesame oil
- 1 teaspoon freshly grated horseradish
- 2 celery ribs, thinly sliced
- 1 scallion, thinly sliced
- 1 tablespoon roasted sesame seeds
- 2 avocados, pitted, peeled, and sliced

Place the seaweeds in a large bowl and add enough cold water to cover by 3 inches. Let stand until just softened, about 10 minutes. Drain well.

Bring a medium saucepan of water to a boil over high heat. Add the shrimp and cook until just opaque throughout, about 3 minutes. Drain and rinse under cold water until cool.

In a separate large bowl, combine the tamari, vinegar, sesame oil, and horseradish and mix well. Stir in the seaweed, celery, scallion, and cooled shrimp. Sprinkle with the sesame seeds.

Divide the salad among four plates, top with the sliced avocado, and serve.

Nutritional analysis per serving: *Calories: 320, Fat: 20 g, Saturated Fat: 3 g, Cholesterol: 145 mg, Fiber: 11 g, Protein: 20 g, Carbohydrates: 18 g, Sodium: 500 mg*

ALMOND CHICKEN SALAD

Radicchio, an Italian lettuce, adds beautiful color to this zesty salad. Radicchio is best when fresh and in season, from January through April. However, most markets carry it year-round, so you shouldn't have any trouble finding it.

- ⅓ cup sliced almonds
- 4 (4-ounce) thin-cut chicken cutlets
- ¼ cup plus 2 tablespoons extra-virgin olive oil
- ½ teaspoon sea salt
- grated zest and juice of 2 limes
- 2 small shallots, minced
- 2 teaspoons chili powder
- 1 teaspoon paprika
- 1 head romaine lettuce, roughly torn
- 1 head radicchio, shredded
- ½ head napa cabbage, shredded
- 2 carrots, peeled and shaved into strips

Serves: 4

Prep Time: 20 minutes

Cook Time: 8 minutes

Preheat the oven to 450°F.

Toast the almonds in a small skillet over medium heat, stirring frequently, until golden brown, 2 to 4 minutes.

Heat a well-seasoned stovetop grill pan over high heat. Rub the chicken cutlets with 2 tablespoons of the oil and season with ¼ teaspoon of the salt. Working in batches, place the chicken on the grill pan and cook for 2 to 3 minutes per side. Transfer the chicken to a cutting board and let cool. Once cool, slice each chicken cutlet into strips.

In a small bowl, whisk together the remaining ¼ cup oil, lime zest and juice, shallots, chili powder, paprika, and remaining ¼ teaspoon salt.

In a large bowl, combine the lettuce, radicchio, cabbage, and carrots and toss with the vinaigrette to coat evenly. Arrange the warm chicken strips over the salad and garnish with toasted almonds. Serve.

Nutritional analysis per serving: *Calories: 435, Fat: 28 g, Saturated Fat: 4 g, Cholesterol: 109 mg, Fiber: 7 g, Protein: 38 g, Carbohydrates: 15 g, Sodium: 534 mg*

CAESAR SALAD WITH GRILLED CHICKEN

This version of Caesar salad uses a hard-boiled egg in the dressing instead of the classic raw egg yolk. The cooked egg whites, diced and added to the salad, add extra protein.

- 4 (4- to 6-ounce) boneless, skinless chicken breasts or thighs
- 2 garlic cloves, 1 thinly sliced and 1 minced
- 5 tablespoons extra-virgin olive oil
- ¼ teaspoon sea salt
- ¼ teaspoon freshly ground black pepper
- 1 large omega-3 egg
- 2 teaspoons Dijon mustard
- ½ teaspoon anchovy paste
- ¼ teaspoon Worcestershire sauce
- 2 tablespoons fresh lemon juice
- 1 head romaine lettuce, cut into 2-inch-wide strips

In a large bowl, combine the chicken, sliced garlic, 1 tablespoon of the olive oil, the salt, and the black pepper. Cover and marinate for at least 15 minutes in the refrigerator.

Put the egg in a small saucepan and add enough cold water to cover by 1 inch. Bring to a boil over medium heat, remove from the heat, and cover. Let stand for 10 minutes. Using a slotted spoon, transfer the egg to a bowl and cover with cold water. When cooled, peel the egg. Separate the yolk from the white. Dice the white and set aside.

In a small bowl, use a fork to mash the egg yolk with the minced garlic, Dijon mustard, anchovy paste, and Worcestershire sauce until well combined. Whisk in the lemon juice. Drizzle in the remaining 4 tablespoons oil, whisking as you drizzle, until the dressing is fully combined.

Heat a well-seasoned stovetop grill pan or grill to medium-high. Grill the chicken until it is firm to the touch and cooked through, about 6 minutes per side (the internal temperature should reach 165°F), turning once during cooking. Transfer the chicken to a cutting board and let rest for 5 minutes. Thinly slice the chicken across the grain.

Place the lettuce in a large bowl, add the dressing, and toss well to coat evenly. Top with the sliced chicken, garnish with the diced egg white, and serve.

Nutritional analysis per serving: *Calories: 330, Fat: 22 g, Saturated Fat: 3 g, Cholesterol: 129 mg, Fiber: 3 g, Protein: 28 g, Carbohydrates: 7 g, Sodium: 428 mg*

CHICKEN SALAD IN ENDIVE CUPS

Serves: 4

Prep Time:
20 minutes

This is a great way to use up leftover cooked chicken. If you don't have any cooked chicken on hand, grill or poach 1 pound of boneless, skinless chicken breasts, cool, then cut into bite-size pieces.

- 1 avocado, peeled and pitted
- ¼ cup fresh parsley leaves, plus extra for garnish
- ¼ cup fresh mint leaves, plus extra for garnish
- ¼ cup fresh lemon juice
- 1 teaspoon anchovy paste
- sea salt and freshly ground black pepper
- 1 pound cooked boneless, skinless chicken breasts, cut into ½-inch cubes
- 4 celery ribs, finely diced
- 1 shallot, finely chopped
- 2 Belgian endives, leaves separated

In a food processor or blender, puree the avocado, parsley, mint, lemon juice, 2 tablespoons of water, anchovy paste, ½ teaspoon salt, and ¼ teaspoon black pepper until smooth. Transfer to a large bowl.

Add the chicken, celery, shallot, a pinch of salt, and ¼ teaspoon black pepper. Fold until well mixed.

To serve, divide the chicken salad among the endive leaves (approximately 10 per person) and garnish with additional parsley and mint.

Nutritional analysis per serving: Calories: 260, Fat: 11 g, Saturated Fat: 1.5 g, Cholesterol: 65 mg, Fiber: 12 g, Protein: 25 g, Carbohydrates: 19 g, Sodium: 550 mg

PAN-ROASTED CHICKEN THIGHS WITH CELERY SALAD AND MUSTARD VINAIGRETTE

Serves: 4

Prep Time:
20 minutes

Cook Time:
20 minutes

Prepare this hearty salad a few hours ahead of time and store it in the refrigerator. The flavors really come together, and the salad only gets better with time.

- 2 anchovy fillets, minced
- 1½ tablespoons fresh lemon juice
- 1 teaspoon Dijon mustard
- 1½ teaspoons celery seeds
- 3 tablespoons extra-virgin olive oil
- 1 pound celery hearts with leaves, thinly sliced
- 10 to 12 radishes (about 8 ounces), julienned
- 3 scallions, chopped
- 1 tablespoon coconut oil
- 1 pound boneless, skinless chicken thighs
- ¼ teaspoon sea salt
- ¼ teaspoon freshly ground black pepper

In a small bowl, combine the minced anchovies, lemon juice, mustard, and 1 teaspoon of the celery seed. Whisk in the olive oil to emulsify the dressing.

In a large bowl, combine the celery, radishes, and scallions. Drizzle the dressing over the salad and toss. Let the salad sit while you make the chicken.

In a large nonstick sauté pan, warm the coconut oil over medium-high heat until shimmering. Season the chicken thighs with the salt and black pepper. Add the chicken to the pan and sauté, turning occasionally, until fully cooked, 16 to 18 minutes, depending on thickness. Cut into one of the thickest chicken thighs to check for doneness; the internal temperature should be 165°F and the juices should run clear. Remove the chicken from the pan and sprinkle with the remaining ½ teaspoon celery seed.

To serve, divide the salad among four plates and top each with a chicken thigh.

Nutritional analysis per serving: *Calories: 280, Fat: 19 g, Saturated Fat: 6 g, Cholesterol: 110 mg, Fiber: 3 g, Protein: 23 g, Carbohydrates: 6 g, Sodium: 400 mg*

WALDORF SALAD WITH SMOKED PAPRIKA

Serves: 4

Prep Time:
30 minutes,
plus chilling
time

Cook Time:
10 minutes

Most commercial mayonnaise on the market is laden with preservatives, additives, and even sweeteners that are not necessary and thus make mayo a junk food. Make your own mayo from organic omega-3 eggs (see page 299; it's easier than you think!) or try Vegenaise, an eggless "mayo" made from canola oil.

- 1 teaspoon dried rosemary
- 1 teaspoon dried thyme
- ½ teaspoon sea salt
- ½ teaspoon freshly ground black pepper
- 1 pound thin-cut chicken cutlets
- 2 large celery ribs with leaves, thinly sliced
- 2 scallions, chopped
- 1 red bell pepper, seeded and chopped
- ½ cup chopped walnuts
- 3 tablespoons Mayonnaise (page 299) or Vegenaise
- 1 tablespoon fresh lemon juice
- 1 teaspoon smoked paprika
- 4 cups mixed salad greens

Fill a skillet with 2 inches of water. Add the rosemary, thyme, and ¼ teaspoon each of the salt and black pepper and bring to a boil over high heat. Add the chicken. Cover, reduce the heat to medium, and cook until done, about 10 minutes. Transfer the chicken cutlets to a bowl and let them cool. Reserve 2 tablespoons of the cooking liquid.

Cut or shred the cooled chicken into small pieces. Add the celery, scallions, bell pepper, and walnuts to the chicken.

In a small bowl, whisk together the reserved poaching liquid, mayonnaise, lemon juice, paprika, and the remaining ¼ teaspoon each salt and black pepper. Add the dressing to the chicken mixture, stirring to combine. Cover and refrigerate for 2 to 3 hours to allow the flavors to mingle.

To serve, divide the salad greens among four plates and top with the chicken salad.

Nutritional analysis per serving: *Calories: 320, Fat: 21 g, Saturated Fat: 2.5 g, Cholesterol: 75 mg, Fiber: 3 g, Protein: 28 g, Carbohydrates: 7 g, Sodium: 510 mg*

TANDOORI LETTUCE CUPS WITH CUMIN SAUCE

Serves: 6

Prep Time:
25 minutes,
plus marinating
time

Cook Time:
20 minutes

This is a hearty meal packed with healing spices that cool inflammation throughout the body. Don't let the lettuce deceive you—you will be energized and satisfied for hours after enjoying this Indian dish.

- 2 tablespoons fresh lemon juice
- 4 scallions, thinly sliced
- 3 tablespoons chopped fresh ginger
- 1 tablespoon paprika
- 2½ teaspoons ground cumin
- ½ teaspoon sea salt
- ¼ teaspoon cayenne pepper
- 2 pounds boneless, skinless chicken thighs, cut into 1½-inch pieces
- 2 to 3 tablespoons extra-virgin olive oil
- 1 red bell pepper, seeded and cut into ½-inch-thick strips
- 1 yellow bell pepper, seeded and cut into ½-inch-thick strips
- 1 small red onion, halved and thinly sliced
- ½ cup Mayonnaise (page 299) or Vegenaise
- grated zest and juice of 1 lime
- 1 small head Boston lettuce, leaves separated
- cilantro sprigs, for garnish

In a large bowl, combine the lemon juice, scallions, ginger, paprika, 2 teaspoons of the cumin, ¼ teaspoon of the salt, and the cayenne and mix well. Add the chicken and toss to coat. Cover and marinate for at least 20 minutes and up to 2½ hours in the refrigerator.

Heat a well-seasoned stovetop grill pan over medium-high heat. Brush with 1 tablespoon of the oil. Remove the chicken from the marinade and grill the chicken, turning occasionally, until no longer pink in the center, 8 to 10 minutes. Work in batches if necessary, adding more oil to the pan if needed. Transfer the cooked chicken to a plate.

Meanwhile, preheat the broiler. On a large rimmed baking sheet, toss the bell peppers and onion with the remaining 1 tablespoon oil. Broil until fork-tender, 12 to 15 minutes, tossing once to ensure even cooking.

In a small bowl, whisk together the mayonnaise, lime zest and juice, remaining ½ teaspoon cumin, and remaining ¼ teaspoon salt.

To serve, have guests wrap chicken and vegetables in lettuce leaves and top with cumin sauce and cilantro sprigs.

Nutritional analysis per serving: *Calories: 400, Fat: 28 g, Saturated Fat: 4.5 g, Cholesterol: 150 mg, Fiber: 1 g, Protein: 30 g, Carbohydrates: 5 g, Sodium: 430 mg*

CHICKEN SATAY WITH CUCUMBER SALAD

Serves: 4

Prep Time:
25 minutes

Cook Time:
15 minutes

Sesame-Coconut Curry Sauce is the perfect accompaniment for these Thai-inspired chicken skewers, and the cucumber salad provides a cool, crisp crunch. You will need eight wooden or bamboo skewers for this recipe; soak them in warm water for at least 15 minutes before cooking so that they don't burn.

- 1 tablespoon Thai fish sauce or gluten-free, low-sodium tamari
- 1 tablespoon plus 2 teaspoons fresh lime juice
- 1 large shallot, minced
- 2 garlic cloves, minced
- 1 teaspoon minced fresh ginger
- ¼ teaspoon ground turmeric
- 1½ pounds boneless, skinless chicken thighs, cut into 1-inch-thick strips
- 8 ounces green beans, trimmed and halved
- 1 small hothouse or English cucumber, peeled, halved lengthwise, and thinly sliced
- ½ small red onion, thinly sliced
- 2 teaspoons extra-virgin olive oil, plus extra if needed for baking sheet
- ¼ teaspoon toasted sesame oil
- ¼ teaspoon sea salt
- Sesame-Coconut Curry Sauce (page 291)

Preheat the oven to 450°F, or heat a grill or well-seasoned stovetop grill pan over medium-high heat.

In a large bowl, whisk together the Thai fish sauce, 1 tablespoon of the lime juice, the shallot, garlic, ginger, and turmeric. Add the chicken and toss to coat. Place the chicken in the refrigerator to marinate for 10 minutes.

Meanwhile, pour 1 cup of water into the bottom of a medium saucepan and bring it to a boil over high heat. Place a steaming rack or basket over the boiling water. Add the green beans, cover, and steam until bright green and crisp-tender, 4 to 5 minutes.

Transfer the green beans to a medium bowl. Add the cucumber, onion, remaining 2 teaspoons lime juice, olive oil, sesame oil, and salt and toss well to combine.

Thread the chicken strips onto the skewers, allowing them to bunch up slightly and covering as much skewer as possible. Leave just the tip and end of the skewers exposed.

If using the oven, lay the skewers on a lightly oiled baking sheet and roast, turning once, until cooked through, 10 to 15 minutes, or grill for 2 to 3 minutes on each side.

Serve the satay with the cucumber salad. Offer the curry sauce alongside for dipping.

Nutritional analysis per serving: *Calories: 260, Fat: 10 g, Saturated Fat: 2 g, Cholesterol: 160 mg, Fiber: 2 g, Protein: 35 g, Carbohydrates: 8 g, Sodium: 575 mg*

THAI CHICKEN SALAD

Serves: 4

Prep Time:
15 minutes

Cook Time:
10 minutes

If you're in a hurry, leftover cooked chicken works great in this salad; just skip the poaching step. The poaching liquid makes a delicious soup base, though. Let it cool and store it in the refrigerator for up to 3 days or in the freezer for up to 6 months.

- 4 cups low-sodium chicken stock
- 8 thin slices peeled ginger
- 3 garlic cloves, halved
- 1 scallion, cut into 2-inch pieces
- ½ teaspoon sea salt
- 2 boneless, skinless chicken breasts, cut into 1-inch pieces
- 2 tablespoons extra-virgin olive oil
- 1 tablespoon fresh lime juice
- 1 tablespoon Thai fish sauce
- pinch of crushed red pepper flakes
- 1 medium head napa or green cabbage, shredded
- ¼ cup thinly sliced red onion or shallot
- 1 cup thinly sliced cucumber
- 4 plum tomatoes, cut into 8 wedges
- ½ cup roughly chopped mixed fresh herbs, such as cilantro, mint, and/or basil
- 2 tablespoons slivered or sliced almonds

In a medium saucepan, combine the chicken stock, ginger, garlic, scallion, and salt. Bring to a gentle simmer over medium heat, then add the chicken. Cover the pan, turn the heat to the lowest setting, and simmer for 8 minutes. Turn off the heat and let the chicken sit in the liquid for 2 more minutes, then transfer the chicken to a plate to cool. (Save the poaching liquid for another use, if desired.)

While the chicken poaches and cools, whisk together the olive oil, lime juice, fish sauce, and red pepper flakes in a large bowl. When the chicken is cool, gently pull it apart into large shreds, add it to the dressing, and toss.

Add the cabbage, onion, cucumber, and tomatoes to the bowl. Toss to combine well. Top with the herbs and almonds and serve.

Nutritional analysis per serving: *Calories: 220, Fat: 12 g, Saturated Fat: 2 g, Cholesterol: 65 mg, Fiber: 2 g, Protein: 21 g, Carbohydrates: 6 g, Sodium: 564 mg*

CHINESE CHICKEN SALAD

Serves: 4

Prep Time:
20 minutes

Cook Time:
20 minutes

This lemon-scented salad brightens the palate and awakens your senses. Choose a lemon with a thin skin, bright yellow color, and a slightly tender touch.

- 1 large head napa cabbage, shredded
- 1 large daikon radish, peeled and grated
- 1 large carrot, peeled and grated
- ½ cup sliced sugar snap peas
- 2 scallions, finely chopped
- 1½ tablespoons extra-virgin olive oil
- 1 tablespoon fresh lemon juice
- 2 teaspoons gluten-free, low-sodium tamari
- ½ teaspoon grated fresh lemon zest
- 4 (4-ounce) boneless, skinless chicken thighs
- ¼ teaspoon sea salt
- ¼ teaspoon freshly ground black pepper
- 1 tablespoon coconut oil
- 1 to 2 teaspoons sesame seeds

In a large bowl, combine the napa cabbage, daikon radish, carrot, sugar snap peas, and scallions. Add the olive oil, lemon juice, tamari, and lemon zest and toss to combine.

Season the chicken with the salt and black pepper. In a large nonstick pan, warm the coconut oil over medium-high heat. Sauté the chicken until golden brown and cooked through (the internal temperature should reach 165°F), 8 to 10 minutes per side.

Divide the salad between four plates and top with the chicken. Garnish with sesame seeds and serve.

Nutritional analysis per serving: Calories: 243, Fat: 14 g, Saturated Fat: 5 g, Cholesterol: 108 mg, Fiber: 2 g, Protein: 24 g, Carbohydrates: 5 g, Sodium: 387 mg

Chicken Yakitori with Napa Cabbage Slaw

Serves: 4

Prep Time: 20 minutes

Cook Time: 10 minutes

Yakitori is simply Japanese for small, bite-size pieces of chicken (or other meat) that have been skewered, marinated, and grilled. Once you try this dish and experience firsthand how simple and tasty this style of cooking can be, you will return to this recipe time and time again. You will need eight wooden or bamboo skewers for this recipe; soak them in warm water for at least 15 minutes before cooking so that they don't burn.

- 1 tablespoon gluten-free, low-sodium tamari
- 2 teaspoons toasted sesame oil
- 2 teaspoons fresh lemon or lime juice
- 1 teaspoon grated fresh ginger
- 1½ pounds boneless, skinless chicken thighs, cut into 1-inch-thick pieces
- 8 ounces green beans, trimmed and halved
- 1 large head napa cabbage, finely shredded
- 4 large radishes, halved and thinly sliced
- 1½ tablespoons extra-virgin olive oil, plus more if needed for baking sheet
- ¼ teaspoon sea salt
- 8 large cremini or button mushrooms, trimmed and quartered
- 1 small zucchini, halved lengthwise and cut crosswise into ¼-inch-thick slices

Preheat the oven to 450°F, or heat a grill or well-seasoned stovetop grill pan over medium-high heat.

In a large bowl, combine the tamari, 1 teaspoon of the sesame oil, 1 teaspoon of the citrus juice, and the ginger and mix well. Add the chicken and place in the refrigerator to marinate for 10 minutes.

Meanwhile, pour 1 cup of water into the bottom of a medium saucepan and bring it to a boil over high heat. Place a steaming rack or basket over the boiling water. Add the green beans, cover, and steam until bright green and crisp-tender, 4 to 5 minutes. Transfer the beans to a large bowl.

Add the cabbage and radishes to the beans, then add 1 tablespoon of the olive oil, the salt, the remaining 1 teaspoon sesame oil, and the remaining 1 teaspoon citrus juice. Toss the slaw well and set aside.

Thread the chicken, mushrooms, and zucchini slices onto the skewers, bunching up the chicken slightly to keep it compact. Try to fill up most of each skewer, leaving only a little wood exposed at each end.

If using the oven, lay the skewers on a lightly oiled baking sheet and brush the mushrooms and zucchini with the remaining ½ tablespoon olive oil. Roast, turning once, until cooked through, about 8 minutes, or grill for 2 to 3 minutes on each side.

Divide the slaw among four plates and serve with two skewers on each.

Nutritional analysis per serving: *Calories: 300, Fat: 13 g, Saturated Fat: 2.5 g, Cholesterol: 160 mg, Fiber: 3 g, Protein: 36 g, Carbohydrates: 9 g, Sodium: 490 mg*

Creamy Berry Smoothie (page 67)

Crustless Asparagus Quiche (page 70)

Vegetable Hash with Fried Eggs (page 71)

Wild Mushroom and Leek Frittata (page 77)

Cherry Tomato and Tofu Salad (page 89)

Brussels Sprouts and Broccoli Slaw with Seared Scallops (page 91)

Niçoise Salad with Poached Salmon (page 100)

Taco Salad with Flank Steak (page 124)

Tomato–Basil Soup with Shrimp (page 128)

Cioppino (page 139)

Fried "Rice" with Shrimp (page 148)

Chipotle Salmon with Arugula Salad (page 160)

Asian-Spiced Salmon Cakes (page 163)

Bok Choy Stir-Fry with Black Cod (page 168)

Miso–Marinated Cod with Fresh Basil and Bok Choy (page 170)

Onion–Leek Soup (page 126)

CHICKEN SPRING ROLLS WITH ALMOND SAUCE

This recipe introduces kelp noodles as an alternative to grain-based pasta. Kelp noodles are made from sea vegetables and are very low in carbohydrates. You can usually find them in the Asian section of your grocery store. If you can't, feel free to use shirataki noodles, which are made from water and glucomannan fiber from the konjac root (you can typically find these in the refrigerated section where other vegetarian foods, such as tofu, tempeh, hummus, and miso, are kept).

- 1½ teaspoons coconut oil
- 1 pound thin-cut chicken cutlets, cut crosswise into strips
- ¼ teaspoon sea salt
- ¼ teaspoon freshly ground black pepper
- ½ cup almond butter
- 1 large scallion, roughly chopped
- 1½ teaspoons coconut amino acids
- ¼ teaspoon ground ginger
- 1½ cups chopped kelp noodles or shirataki noodles
- 16 fresh mint leaves
- 16 Boston or butter lettuce leaves
- ¼ small red onion, thinly sliced
- ½ medium daikon radish, peeled and julienned
- 1 medium red bell pepper, seeded and thinly sliced
- ½ cup sliced hearts of palm, drained if canned

In a large nonstick sauté pan, warm the coconut oil over medium-high heat. Season the chicken with the salt and black pepper and add to the pan. Cook until the chicken is cooked through, about 2 minutes per side.

In a food processor, combine the almond butter, scallion, amino acids, and ginger. Process, adding 4 to 5 tablespoons of hot water through the feed tube until the sauce reaches the desired consistency.

Place the noodles in a colander and rinse well. In a small bowl, mix the noodles with about half of the almond sauce, reserving the remaining sauce.

To make the spring rolls, place a mint leaf at the bottom of each lettuce leaf. Add a small amount of noodles, chicken, onion, daikon, bell pepper, and hearts of palm. Top with a tablespoon of almond sauce. Repeat to make the remaining rolls. Serve.

Nutritional analysis per serving: *Calories: 410, Fat: 23 g, Saturated Fat: 4.5 g, Cholesterol: 75 mg, Fiber: 6 g, Protein: 33 g, Carbohydrates: 20 g, Sodium: 480 mg*

Fennel and Cherry Tomato Salad with Pork Tenderloin

Choose pasture-raised, grass-fed pork from your local market, when possible, to avoid antibiotics typically used for animals raised in confinement. In moderation, pork can be a delicious protein source you can feel good about enjoying. As with all meat, balance, variety, and moderation are key.

- 2 medium fennel bulbs, quartered and thinly sliced, plus 2 tablespoons chopped fennel fronds
- 2 pints cherry tomatoes, halved
- 1 cup julienned jicama
- 1 large scallion, finely chopped
- 1 teaspoon fennel seeds
- 2½ tablespoons extra-virgin olive oil
- 1 tablespoon fresh lemon juice
- sea salt and freshly ground black pepper
- ½ teaspoon dried rosemary
- 1 (1-pound) pork tenderloin, cut into bite-size pieces

In a large bowl, combine the fennel slices and fronds, tomatoes, jicama, scallion, fennel seeds, 2 tablespoons of the olive oil, the lemon juice, ¼ teaspoon salt, and a pinch of black pepper. Stir to combine.

Meanwhile, in a spice grinder, pulse the rosemary, ¼ teaspoon salt, and a pinch of black pepper. Firmly rub the pork tenderloin pieces with the rosemary seasoning.

Warm the remaining ½ tablespoon olive oil in a large nonstick pan over medium-high heat. Add the pork and sauté, stirring occasionally, until the pork is cooked through, 5 to 6 minutes.

Transfer the pork to the salad. Stir to combine and serve.

Nutritional analysis per serving: *Calories: 280, Fat: 15 g, Saturated Fat: 3 g, Cholesterol: 60 mg, Fiber: 7 g, Protein: 22 g, Carbohydrates: 18 g, Sodium: 420 mg*

TACO SALAD WITH FLANK STEAK

Serves: 4

Prep Time:
20 minutes

Cook Time:
15 minutes

The coriander and cayenne make this dish pop. Coriander is a slightly sweet spice and the cayenne has a nice amount of heat—both complement the citrus in this steak salad and make you feel as though you are at a Mexican fiesta.

- 1 bunch cilantro, including stems
- 1 scallion, thinly sliced
- ¼ cup extra-virgin olive oil
- 2 tablespoons Mayonnaise (page 299) or Vegenaise
- 2 teaspoons white vinegar
- grated zest and juice of ½ lime
- sea salt and freshly ground black pepper
- 1 (1-pound) grass-fed flank steak
- 1 teaspoon ground coriander
- ½ teaspoon cayenne pepper
- 2 large romaine lettuce hearts, halved lengthwise and thinly sliced
- 1 pint cherry or grape tomatoes, halved
- 4 medium bell peppers (any color), seeded and thinly sliced into rings
- 1 avocado, pitted, peeled, and thinly sliced
- 2 tablespoons toasted pepitas
- lime wedges, for serving

In a blender, combine the cilantro, 1 teaspoon of the sliced scallion, the olive oil, mayonnaise, vinegar, lime zest and juice, 2 tablespoons of water, ½ teaspoon salt, and a pinch of black pepper. Puree until very smooth, 1 to 2 minutes, and set aside.

Heat a well-seasoned stovetop grill pan over medium-high heat. Season the steak with ¼ teaspoon salt and ½ teaspoon black pepper. When the pan is very hot, cook the steak until charred, turning once, 12 to 15 minutes for medium-rare (about 135°F). Transfer the steak to a cutting board and immediately sprinkle both sides with the coriander and cayenne. Let stand for 10 minutes, then cut into bite-size pieces.

In a large bowl, toss the romaine with one-third of the dressing and divide among four plates. Arrange the tomatoes, bell peppers, avocado, and steak on top and drizzle with the remaining dressing. Sprinkle the pepitas and remaining sliced scallion on top. Serve with lime wedges on the side.

Nutritional analysis per serving: *Calories: 468, Fat: 32 g, Saturated Fat: 6 g, Cholesterol: 72 mg, Fiber: 8 g, Protein: 30 g, Carbohydrates: 18 g, Sodium: 526 mg*

ONION-LEEK SOUP

Serves: 4

Prep Time:
15 minutes

Cook Time:
20 minutes

If you can't find chervil, you can substitute ¾ cup chopped fresh parsley plus ¼ cup chopped fresh tarragon. To make this a vegetarian soup, simply replace the chicken stock with vegetable stock (such as the Vegetable–Herb Stock on page 304).

- 2 tablespoons extra-virgin olive oil, plus more for serving
- 3 leeks, white parts only, halved lengthwise and thinly sliced crosswise
- 1 medium yellow onion, quartered and very thinly sliced
- ¾ teaspoon sea salt
- ½ teaspoon freshly ground black pepper
- 4 cups low-sodium chicken stock
- 1 (14-ounce) package non-GMO silken tofu, drained and quartered
- 1 cup chopped fresh chervil, plus more for garnish
- 2 tablespoons chopped toasted almonds

Heat the oil in a large saucepan over medium heat. Add the leeks and onion and season with ½ teaspoon salt and ¼ teaspoon black pepper. Stir well and cover. Cook, stirring occasionally, until translucent, about 5 minutes.

Add the stock to the saucepan. Bring to a boil, then reduce the heat to low, and simmer, uncovered, until the leeks are very soft, about 10 minutes. Add the tofu and return to a boil. Turn off the heat and carefully transfer the soup to a blender (see Note). Add the chervil and the remaining ¼ teaspoon each salt and black pepper and blend until very smooth, 2 to 3 minutes. (Alternatively, you can use an immersion blender to puree the soup right in the pan.)

Ladle the soup into four serving bowls and top each serving with chervil and almonds.

Note: Always be very careful when pureeing hot liquids in a blender. The heat from the liquid can cause the pressure in the blender to build up under the lid, and when the blender is turned on, the top can blow off and your hot soup will fly everywhere. Keep the lid vented by removing the small window insert from the middle of the blender lid; hold a towel over the open window to prevent splattering. Always start on the lowest speed possible.

Nutritional analysis per serving: *Calories: 290, Fat: 13 g, Saturated Fat: 2 g, Cholesterol: 25 mg, Fiber: 5 g, Protein: 14 g, Carbohydrates: 31 g, Sodium: 600 mg*

Tomato-Basil Soup with Shrimp

Serves: 4

Prep Time:
10 minutes

Cook Time:
30 minutes

One of my favorite culinary tricks for making creamy, comforting soups without dairy is substituting cashews for heavy cream or butter in recipes. Cashews are mild in flavor and lend a creaminess that you can't get from other nuts. They also happen to be quite hypoallergenic, which is helpful for those with tree nut allergies.

- 1 cup raw cashews
- 2 tablespoons extra-virgin olive oil
- 1 yellow onion, diced
- 4 garlic cloves, sliced
- 1 celery rib, diced
- 1 bay leaf
- 1 tablespoon tomato paste
- 1 (28-ounce) can tomato puree
- 1½ cups low-sodium chicken stock
- ¼ cup unsweetened almond milk
- ½ teaspoon sea salt
- ¼ cup tightly packed fresh basil leaves, plus extra chopped basil for garnish
- 20 large cooked, peeled shrimp
- freshly ground black pepper

Place the cashews in a small, heatproof bowl and cover with 2 cups of boiling water. Cover the bowl and allow the cashews to sit for 15 minutes, then drain and reserve the nuts.

While the cashews are soaking, heat the olive oil in a medium saucepan over medium heat. Add the onion, garlic, celery, and bay leaf to the pan and cook, stirring occasionally, until the vegetables are soft and beginning to brown, about 10 minutes.

Stir in the tomato paste and cook for 2 more minutes. Add the tomato puree, chicken stock, almond milk, cashews, and salt. Bring to a simmer, then reduce the heat to medium-low and cook for 15 minutes.

Remove the bay leaf and transfer the hot soup to a blender, and very carefully puree the soup starting on low speed, making sure to vent the lid (see Note). Once the soup is pureed, add the basil and give it a quick final spin in the blender.

Divide the shrimp among four soup bowls and ladle the soup into each bowl. Sprinkle a pinch of black pepper over each bowl of soup, garnish with chopped basil, and serve.

Note: Always be very careful when pureeing hot liquids in a blender. The heat from the liquid can cause the pressure in the blender to build up under the lid, and when the blender is turned on, the top can blow off and your hot soup will fly everywhere. Keep the lid vented by removing the small window insert from the middle of the blender lid; hold a towel over the open window to prevent splattering. Always start on the lowest speed possible.

Nutritional analysis per serving: *Calories: 360, Fat: 21 g, Saturated Fat: 3.5 g, Cholesterol: 55 mg, Fiber: 6 g, Protein: 16 g, Carbohydrates: 32 g, Sodium: 490 mg*

Thai Chicken Noodle Soup

Serves: 4

Prep Time:
15 minutes

Cook Time:
20 minutes

Kelp noodles are simple to prepare and low-glycemic. Their neutral flavor makes them an easy, versatile addition to soups such as this one. For a more substantial meal, pair this with Arugula and Fennel Salad (see page 252).

- 4 cups low-sodium chicken stock
- 1 (13.5-ounce) can full-fat unsweetened coconut milk
- 1 yellow onion, quartered and thinly sliced
- 2 lemongrass stalks, cut into 4-inch lengths and smashed
- 1 long red chile (such as Anaheim), seeded and thinly sliced
- 1 pound boneless, skinless chicken breasts, cut into strips
- 1 cup halved sugar snap peas
- 1 pound kelp noodles, rinsed and drained
- 3 ounces bean sprouts
- ½ teaspoon sea salt
- ½ bunch cilantro, including stems, chopped
- lime wedges, for serving

Combine the chicken stock, coconut milk, and 1½ cups of water in a large stockpot. Add the onion, lemongrass, and chile and bring to a boil over medium-high heat. Reduce the heat to low and simmer until the onion is translucent, about 10 minutes.

Add the chicken and sugar snap peas and poach until the chicken is just cooked through, about 5 minutes. Discard the lemongrass. Add the kelp noodles and bean sprouts and cook until the noodles are just soft, about 2 minutes. Stir in the salt.

Divide the soup among four serving bowls and top with the cilantro. Serve with the lime wedges.

Nutritional analysis per serving: *Calories: 440, Fat: 25 g, Saturated Fat: 19 g, Cholesterol: 100 mg, Fiber: 4 g, Protein: 35 g, Carbohydrates: 21 g, Sodium: 490 mg*

DINNER
Vegetarian and Vegan

Broccoli Tofu

It seems wherever I go, people ask me whether broccoli is good for thyroid health. When you cook broccoli just enough, you remove the goitrogenic compounds called thiocyanates. While thiocyanates are important for disease prevention and overall health, there is no research showing that they interfere with thyroid health. This recipe is one of my favorite ways to show people how to prepare broccoli for nutritional health as well as flavor and enjoyment.

- 2 (14-ounce) packages non-GMO extra-firm tofu
- 1 teaspoon sea salt
- 1½ pounds broccoli, stems peeled and cut into ¼-inch-thick rounds, florets separated into bite-size pieces
- 4 tablespoons extra-virgin olive oil
- ¼ cup gluten-free, low-sodium tamari
- ¼ teaspoon crushed red pepper flakes
- 4 garlic cloves, thinly sliced
- 1 (8-ounce) can sliced water chestnuts, drained
- ½ cup coarsely chopped roasted cashews

Serves: 6

Prep Time: 20 minutes, plus draining time

Cook Time: 15 minutes

Drain the tofu by placing the two blocks of tofu side by side on a rimmed baking sheet lined with several layers of paper towels. Top with additional paper towels and another baking sheet, and set something heavy, such as some canned goods, on the top baking sheet to help press out the liquid. Allow the tofu to drain for at least 30 minutes, changing the paper towels at least once. Cut the tofu into 1-inch cubes and set aside. Discard the wet paper towels from the baking sheet and apply new dry ones; set aside.

Bring a 5-quart pot of water to a boil over high heat. Add ½ teaspoon of the salt. Cook the broccoli stems and florets until bright green, 1 to

2 minutes. Drain the broccoli in a colander and rinse with cold water, tossing until cool. Dry thoroughly and set aside.

In a large nonstick skillet, heat 2 tablespoons of the oil over medium-high heat until shimmering. Add the tofu and cook until golden brown, 2 to 3 minutes on each side. Once the tofu is browned, transfer it to the lined baking sheet. Reserve the oil in the pan.

In a small bowl whisk together the tamari, ¼ cup of water, the red pepper flakes, and the remaining ½ teaspoon salt and set aside.

Add the remaining 2 tablespoons oil to the skillet and heat over high heat until shimmering. Add the broccoli, garlic, and water chestnuts and cook for 5 to 7 minutes, tossing often to avoid burning the garlic. Whisk the tamari sauce again and add it to the pan, along with the tofu, and toss to coat as the sauce thickens, about 1 minute more. Serve, topped with cashews.

Nutritional analysis per serving: Calories: 330, Fat: 22 g, Saturated Fat: 3.5 g, Cholesterol: 0 mg, Fiber: 6 g, Protein: 20 g, Carbohydrates: 16 g, Sodium: 432 mg

Roasted Vegetable Lasagna with Cashew "Ricotta"

Serves: 6

Prep Time:
30 minutes

Cook Time:
55 minutes

Who says you can't enjoy comfort food while nourishing your body? Prepare this dish when you want to share a hearty, delicious meal the entire family will love. From my experience, it is best to double the recipe, making two lasagnas and freezing one for later, because this will quickly become a family favorite!

- 1 small eggplant, very thinly sliced lengthwise
- 1 zucchini, very thinly sliced lengthwise
- 1 yellow summer squash, very thinly sliced lengthwise
- 1 bell pepper (any color), seeded and cut into large squares
- ¼ cup extra-virgin olive oil
- 1 teaspoon sea salt
- 2 cups Cashew "Ricotta Cheese" (page 295)
- 1 large omega-3 egg, beaten
- ½ teaspoon dried oregano
- pinch of freshly ground black pepper
- 1 (15-ounce) can crushed tomatoes

Preheat the oven to 400°F.

In a large bowl, combine the eggplant, zucchini, summer squash, and bell pepper with the oil and salt and toss well. Spread the vegetables in a single layer on two baking sheets and roast until they start to brown and caramelize around the edges, 20 to 25 minutes, rotating the sheets halfway through the cooking time.

Remove the baking sheets from the oven and set them aside to cool. Lower the oven temperature to 350°F.

While the vegetables are cooling, whisk together the cashew "cheese," egg, oregano, and black pepper in a medium bowl. Spread one-fourth of the mixture in the bottom of a 9-inch square glass baking dish, then spoon ½ cup of the crushed tomatoes on top. Cover the tomatoes with a layer of one of the types of vegetables. Continue to layer the remaining

133

"cheese," tomatoes, and vegetables until everything is used up, finishing with tomatoes.

Bake the lasagna for 30 minutes. Allow it to cool for 5 minutes before serving.

Nutritional analysis per serving: *Calories: 440, Fat: 34 g, Saturated Fat: 6 g, Cholesterol: 40 mg, Fiber: 6 g, Protein: 12 g, Carbohydrates: 28 g, Sodium: 512 mg*

Coconut Curry with Tofu

The jalapeños make this curry nice and spicy. For a milder version, use only 2 jalapeños, and remove the seeds.

- 1 small bunch cilantro
- grated zest of 1 lime
- 3 jalapeños, seeded if desired
- 2 garlic cloves, halved
- 1 (1-inch) piece ginger, peeled and roughly chopped
- 1 teaspoon ground coriander
- 1 teaspoon sea salt
- ½ teaspoon freshly ground black pepper
- ½ teaspoon ground cumin
- 1 (13.5-ounce) can full-fat unsweetened coconut milk, chilled in the refrigerator overnight or for 12 hours
- 1 (14-ounce) package non-GMO firm tofu, drained and cut into ½-inch cubes
- ½ small head cabbage, cut into 1-inch pieces
- 1 large head broccoli, florets cut into 1-inch pieces
- 1 large head cauliflower, cored, florets cut into ½-inch pieces
- lime wedges, for serving

Trim the cilantro leaves from the stems and reserve the leaves for garnish. Put the stems in a food processor and add the lime zest, jalapeños, garlic, ginger, coriander, ½ teaspoon of the salt, the black pepper, and the cumin. Pulse, scraping the sides of the bowl occasionally, until a smooth green curry paste forms.

Spoon 3 tablespoons of thick cream from the top of the can of coconut milk into a large saucepan. Cook over medium heat, stirring, until the oil separates and sizzles, about 1 minute. Add the green curry paste and cook, stirring, until thickened and nearly dry, about 2 minutes. Add the remaining coconut milk and 1 cup of water. Bring to a boil. Add the tofu and return to a boil, then reduce the heat to low and simmer for about 20 minutes.

Meanwhile, bring a large saucepan of water to a boil. Add ¼ teaspoon of the salt to the water. Add the cabbage and cook until the thick white parts are just tender, about 3 minutes. Transfer the cabbage to the curry with a slotted spoon. Add the broccoli and cauliflower to the boiling water. Cook until crisp-tender, about 4 minutes. Drain and add to the curry, along with the remaining ¼ teaspoon salt. Stir well to combine.

Serve the curry, garnished with the reserved cilantro leaves, and lime wedges on the side.

Nutritional analysis per serving: *Calories: 380, Fat: 26 g, Saturated Fat: 19 g, Cholesterol: 0 mg, Fiber: 9 g, Protein: 19 g, Carbohydrates: 26 g, Sodium: 440 mg*

Seafood

Pacific Coast Bouillabaisse

Serves: 6

Prep Time:
30 minutes

Cook Time:
50 minutes

A bouquet garni consists of a variety of herb sprigs bundled together with some kitchen string. It is used to flavor broths, soups, and sauces. The bouquet is removed prior to serving.

- 1 pound firm, lean fish fillets (such as cod, halibut, or bass), cut into 2-inch chunks
- ½ cup extra-virgin olive oil, plus more for drizzling
- sea salt and freshly ground black pepper
- 12 clams, scrubbed
- 2 small yellow onions, chopped
- 2 leeks, chopped, white parts only
- 4 garlic cloves, minced
- 1 (28-ounce) can diced tomatoes
- 1 tablespoon tomato paste
- 4 cups vegetable stock
- 1 bouquet garni (4 parsley sprigs, 1 bay leaf, 1 thyme sprig, 1 strip orange peel, all tied together with kitchen string)
- pinch of saffron
- 1 pound scallops or tender, mild fish fillets (such as snapper or sole) cut into 2-inch chunks
- juice of 1 lime
- chopped fresh tarragon, for garnish

Coat the firm fish chunks with a light drizzle of olive oil and season with a pinch each of salt and black pepper. Cover and chill until ready to use.

Put the clams in a medium saucepan, add 1 cup of water, cover, and heat over medium–high heat just until all of the shells have opened, about 3 minutes. Remove the pan from the heat and set aside, covered.

In a large, nonreactive saucepan, heat the ½ cup oil over medium-low heat until shimmering. Add the onions and leeks with a pinch of salt, and cook until softened but not browned, 8 to 10 minutes. Add the garlic and cook until fragrant, 30 seconds to 1 minute. Add the tomatoes with their juices, tomato paste, vegetable stock, bouquet garni, saffron, and another pinch each of salt and black pepper. Simmer for 20 minutes, then remove and discard the bouquet garni.

Transfer the clams to a bowl and strain their cooking liquid through a fine-mesh sieve to remove any sand particles. Add the strained liquid to the soup. Raise the heat to medium-high and bring the soup to a rapid boil. Gently stir in the firm fish, cover, and let cook for 3 to 4 minutes. Add the scallops or tender fish and cook until just opaque, about 3 minutes. Add the clams and bring back to a simmer for 5 minutes, then turn off the heat (be sure to toss any unopened clams).

Add lime juice to taste. Ladle into soup bowls, garnish with fresh tarragon, and serve.

Nutritional analysis per serving: *Calories: 390, Fat: 22 g, Saturated Fat: 3.5 g, Cholesterol: 70 mg, Fiber: 3 g, Protein: 36 g, Carbohydrates: 14 g, Sodium: 390 mg*

CIOPPINO

Cioppino is a seafood stew with its roots in the fishing community of San Francisco. This version uses flounder, squid, and shrimp, but you can also add mussels or small clams in their shells, crabmeat, or even lobster. Cooking times for fish and shellfish vary, so always add the heartier shellfish to the pan first—allowing their shells to open if using clams or mussels or for their flesh to turn opaque for crabs and lobsters—then follow with shrimp and squid and, finally, the most delicate fish fillets.

- ¼ cup extra-virgin olive oil
- 1 teaspoon fennel seeds
- ½ teaspoon dried oregano
- ¼ teaspoon crushed red pepper flakes, or to taste
- 1 yellow onion, thinly sliced
- 1 small leek, white and light green sections halved lengthwise and thinly sliced
- 2 garlic cloves, thinly sliced
- 1 fennel bulb, thinly sliced
- 1 tablespoon tomato paste
- 1 (28-ounce) can diced tomatoes
- 1 (8-ounce) bottle clam juice
- sea salt and freshly ground black pepper
- 1 pound medium shrimp, peeled and deveined
- 1 pound flounder or other white fish fillet, cut into 2-inch pieces
- 8 ounces squid, bodies sliced into thin rings and tentacles halved lengthwise
- chopped fresh basil, for garnish

Warm the olive oil in a large sauté pan or Dutch oven over low heat. Add the fennel seed, oregano, and red pepper flakes and cook until fragrant, about 2 minutes. Be careful not to burn the spices.

Raise the heat to medium-low and add the onion, leek, garlic, and fennel. Sauté until the vegetables are very soft and just beginning to brown, 7 to 10 minutes.

Add the tomato paste and sauté for 30 seconds, then add the diced tomatoes with their juices (if you prefer a thicker soup, drain the juices) and the clam juice. Bring to a simmer, then lower the heat and cook for 15 minutes, stirring occasionally. Season with ½ teaspoon salt and a pinch of black pepper.

Add the shrimp to the soup and cook just until they begin to turn pink and curl, about 2 minutes. Add the flounder and squid and cook gently, just until they turn white and opaque, about 3 minutes.

Ladle the cioppino into bowls, garnish with basil, and serve.

Nutritional analysis per serving: *Calories: 250, Fat: 12 g, Saturated Fat: 2 g, Cholesterol: 170 mg, Fiber: 2 g, Protein: 27 g, Carbohydrates: 13 g, Sodium: 500 mg*

MONKFISH TAGINE

Serves: 4

Prep Time:
15 minutes

Cook Time:
35 minutes

Tagine refers to both a clay pot used to cook stews in and the stew itself. The pots are very earthy and calming—much like the food they are used to cook. Tagines typically have warming spices and complex flavors from herbs, spices, and vegetables. But you don't need a clay pot to cook this dish; you'll get the same delicious, comforting results without it.

- 1½ teaspoons coconut oil
- 2 medium yellow onions, halved and sliced
- 1 medium fennel bulb, halved and sliced
- 1 teaspoon grated fresh ginger
- 1 teaspoon ground cumin
- ½ teaspoon ground cinnamon
- ½ teaspoon ground coriander
- ½ teaspoon sweet paprika
- sea salt and freshly ground black pepper
- 1¼ cups low-sodium chicken stock
- 1 (8-ounce) can crushed tomatoes, strained
- 1 small cauliflower, cored and cut into 2-inch florets
- 1 pint cherry tomatoes, halved
- ⅓ cup halved Kalamata olives
- 4 (6- to 8-ounce) monkfish fillets
- 2 tablespoons chopped fresh parsley

In a large sauté pan, heat the coconut oil over medium-high heat until shimmering. Add the onions and fennel and sauté until softened, about 10 minutes.

Stir in the ginger, cumin, cinnamon, coriander, paprika, ¼ teaspoon salt, and a pinch of black pepper. Add the chicken stock, strained tomatoes, and cauliflower and stir well. Reduce the heat to medium-low and let the mixture simmer, stirring occasionally, until the cauliflower is somewhat softened, about 10 minutes.

Stir in the cherry tomatoes and olives. Season the monkfish with a pinch of salt and ¼ teaspoon black pepper. Using a wooden spoon, make four little vegetable "nests" and lay a monkfish fillet in each. Cover the pan and let the fish simmer until it is fully cooked and tender, 12 to 15 minutes.

Serve, garnished with parsley.

Nutritional analysis per serving: *Calories: 300, Fat: 9 g, Saturated Fat: 2 g, Cholesterol: 45 mg, Fiber: 8 g, Protein: 31 g, Carbohydrates: 25 g, Sodium: 530 g*

THAI GREEN CURRY WITH SOFT-SHELL CRABS

Serves: 4

Prep Time:
20 minutes

Cook Time:
40 minutes

A favorite culinary trick is dredging or coating your meat in flour and egg to create a crisp, delicious crust. This recipe uses coconut flour instead of white flour, which is high–glycemic and inflammatory.

- 1 tablespoon extra-virgin olive oil
- 1 pound carrots, peeled and cut into 1-inch pieces
- 2 heads baby bok choy, stems cut into 1-inch pieces, leaves reserved
- 1 yellow onion, chopped
- ¼ cup Thai Green Curry Paste (page 302)
- 1 (13.5-ounce) can full-fat unsweetened coconut milk
- 3 large omega-3 egg whites
- 1½ cups coconut flour
- ¼ teaspoon sea salt
- 8 soft-shell crabs, cleaned
- ½ cup grapeseed oil
- 5 ounces baby spinach
- grated zest and juice of 2 limes

Preheat the oven to 250°F.

In a 5–quart Dutch oven, heat the olive oil over medium heat until shimmering. Add the carrots, bok choy stems, and onion. Cook until the onion is translucent, 7 to 10 minutes. Add the curry paste and cook, stirring, until fragrant and blended with the vegetables, about 1 minute.

Add the coconut milk and 3 cups of water, bring to a boil, and then reduce the heat to a simmer. Cook until the carrots are crisp-tender, 8 to 10 minutes. Cover the Dutch oven and transfer it to the bottom rack of the oven to keep warm.

Line two baking sheets with a few layers of paper towels.

Whisk the egg whites until soft peaks form; transfer to a shallow bowl. Fill another shallow bowl with coconut flour and the sea salt. Dip one crab into the egg whites, allowing the excess to drip off. Then dip it into the coconut flour, gently patting it to adhere. Carefully place the crab on one of the lined baking sheets. Repeat with the remaining crabs.

In a large cast-iron skillet, warm the grapeseed oil over medium heat until shimmering, 5 to 7 minutes. The end of a crab leg dipped in the oil will bubble when the oil is ready.

Depending on the size of your skillet, gently place 1 or 2 crabs, shell-side down, in the oil. Cook until the shell is pink and the batter has browned, 2 to 3 minutes. Using a thin metal spatula, gently turn the crabs and continue to cook until brown on the bottom, another 1 to 2 minutes. Transfer to the second lined baking sheet and place in the warm oven. Repeat with the remaining crabs.

Remove the Dutch oven from the oven and stir in the spinach and bok choy leaves. Add the lime zest and juice and stir to combine. Divide the curry among four plates and top each with 2 crabs. Serve.

Nutritional analysis per serving: Calories: 425, Fat: 28 g, Saturated Fat: 21 g, Cholesterol: 74 mg, Fiber: 12 g, Protein: 15 g, Carbohydrates: 36 g, Sodium: 588 mg

TANDOORI SHRIMP WITH INDIAN-SPICED CABBAGE

Serves: 4

Prep Time:
15 minutes, plus marinating time

Cook Time:
20 minutes

Mustard seeds offer a pungent flavor that can be used to enhance curries and stir-fries. The seeds come from the mustard plant, which is from the same family of plants as cruciferous vegetables such as broccoli and cauliflower. Mustard seeds are acclaimed for their health benefits, ranging from reducing high blood pressure and menopausal symptoms to preventing cancer and calming autoimmune disease. There are a variety of mustard seeds—white, yellow, brown, and black. Yellow and brown are the most common in the West, while black seeds are traditionally used in Indian cuisine. You can find mustard seeds in the spice aisle or Asian section of your supermarket, and you can also order them online.

- 2 teaspoons sweet paprika
- 1 teaspoon ground ginger
- 1 teaspoon ground cumin
- 1 teaspoon ground coriander
- 1 teaspoon ground turmeric
- 1 teaspoon mild chili powder
- 1¼ teaspoons sea salt
- ¼ teaspoon cayenne pepper
- ½ cup full-fat unsweetened coconut milk
- 2 tablespoons fresh lime juice
- 1½ pounds large or jumbo shrimp, peeled and deveined
- 4 to 5 tablespoons grapeseed or coconut oil
- ½ teaspoon yellow or brown mustard seeds
- ½ teaspoon fennel seeds
- 1 red onion, thinly sliced
- 1 tablespoon minced fresh ginger
- 1 tablespoon minced garlic
- ½ head cabbage (any kind), shredded
- 1 scallion, thinly sliced
- ¼ cup chopped fresh cilantro, for garnish
- lime wedges, for serving

Create the Tandoori spice mix by combining the paprika, ground ginger, cumin, coriander, turmeric, chili powder, 1 teaspoon salt, and the cayenne pepper in a small bowl.

In a medium bowl, combine the coconut milk, lime juice, and 2 tablespoons of the Tandoori spice mix and mix well. (The leftover spice mix can be stored in an airtight container.) Add the shrimp and toss to coat. Marinate at room temperature for 30 minutes or in the refrigerator, covered, for up to 8 hours.

When you are ready to cook, heat 2 tablespoons of the oil in a large sauté pan over medium heat until shimmering. Add the mustard and fennel seeds and cook just until the mustard seeds start to pop, about 1 minute. Add the onion, minced ginger, and garlic to the pan and sauté until soft and fragrant, about 2 minutes.

Add the cabbage and remaining ¼ teaspoon salt to the pan, turn the heat to high, and sauté the cabbage until it becomes soft and begins to brown, about 10 minutes. You may need to add another tablespoon of oil if the pan seems too dry. (As the cabbage cooks, you can add a few tablespoons of water as needed to release any ingredients that stick to the bottom of the pan.) Transfer the cabbage mixture to a serving platter and stir in the scallion.

Wash and dry the sauté pan and return it to the stove over high heat. Add the remaining 2 tablespoons oil and heat until shimmering. Drain the shrimp from the marinade and reserve any remaining marinade. Using tongs, add the shrimp to the hot oil a few at a time. Sauté the shrimp quickly, just until they turn pink and begin to curl, 4 to 5 minutes. You may have to work in batches to avoid overcrowding the pan. As the shrimp are cooked, place them on top of the cabbage.

Once all of the shrimp are cooked, pour any remaining marinade into the pan and cook for 30 seconds, stirring. Pour the cooked marinade over the shrimp and cabbage. Garnish with the cilantro and serve with lime wedges.

Nutritional analysis per serving: *Calories: 315, Fat: 16 g, Saturated Fat: 2 g, Cholesterol: 274 mg, Fiber: 3 g, Protein: 36 g, Carbohydrates: 8 g, Sodium: 563 mg*

SHRIMP AND THREE-MUSHROOM SAUTÉ WITH CHIVES

Make this meal for lunch or dinner anytime you want something fast yet satisfying and delicious.

- 1½ tablespoons coconut oil
- 1½ pounds medium shrimp, peeled and deveined
- sea salt and freshly ground black pepper
- 4 medium portobello mushroom caps, cut into 1-inch slices
- 7 ounces oyster mushrooms, sliced
- 1½ ounces shiitake mushroom caps, sliced
- 5 ounces baby spinach
- 1 cup snow peas
- 1 large bunch chives, cut into 2-inch pieces
- 1½ teaspoons minced fresh ginger
- 1½ teaspoons coconut amino acids

Serves: 4

Prep Time:
20 minutes

Cook Time:
15 minutes

In a wok or large nonstick sauté pan, heat ½ tablespoon of the oil over high heat until shimmering. Add the shrimp, ¼ teaspoon salt, and a pinch of black pepper and, stirring constantly, sauté until fully cooked, 4 to 5 minutes. Transfer the shrimp to a large bowl.

Add another ½ tablespoon of the oil to the pan and reduce the heat to medium-high. Add the portobello slices and sauté, stirring frequently, until just softened, 4 to 5 minutes. Add the oyster and shiitake mushrooms and cook until softened, 2 to 3 minutes. Transfer the mushrooms to the bowl with the shrimp.

Raise the heat to high and add the remaining ½ tablespoon oil. Add the spinach and snow peas, sautéing until the spinach is wilted, 1 to 2 minutes. Stir in the chives, ginger, and amino acids and cook until the chives are wilted, about 1 minute. Transfer the vegetable mixture to the bowl with the shrimp and mushrooms, stir to combine, and serve.

Nutritional analysis per serving: *Calories: 250, Fat: 7 g, Saturated Fat: 4.5 g, Cholesterol: 275 mg, Fiber: 4 g, Protein: 39 g, Carbohydrates: 11 g, Sodium: 430 mg*

FRIED "RICE" WITH SHRIMP

Serves: 4

Prep Time:
30 minutes

Cook Time:
15 minutes

This recipe is a fun alternative to classic fried rice. By replacing the traditional rice with cauliflower, you gain lots of healthy benefits—try it!

- 1 medium head cauliflower
- 2 teaspoons grapeseed oil
- 2 red bell peppers, seeded and sliced
- 8 ounces snow peas
- 1 (5-ounce) can water chestnuts, drained
- ½ cup raw cashews
- 3 large omega-3 eggs
- 2 cups mung bean sprouts
- 1 pound large shrimp, peeled and deveined
- 1 tablespoon toasted sesame oil
- 3 scallions, chopped, green and white parts separated
- 2 teaspoons minced garlic
- 2 teaspoons minced fresh ginger
- 1 teaspoon gluten-free, low-sodium tamari
- ¼ teaspoon freshly ground black pepper

Cut the cauliflower in half. Place a box grater over a large bowl and grate each cauliflower half over the big holes of the grater—hold the stem of the cauliflower as you grate. Aim for 4 cups of cauliflower "rice."

In a wok or a large sauté pan, heat 1 teaspoon of the grapeseed oil over high heat until shimmering. Cook the red bell peppers for 1 minute; then, add the snow peas, water chestnuts, and cashews and cook until the vegetables are mostly tender, about 4 minutes.

Meanwhile, in a small bowl, whisk the eggs with 1 tablespoon of water. When the vegetables are tender, push them to the side of the pan. Add the eggs, stirring until scrambled, about 1 minute. Stir in the bean sprouts. Transfer the vegetable mixture to a large serving bowl.

Add the remaining 1 teaspoon grapeseed oil to the pan. Add the shrimp and sauté until they are pink and fully cooked, 4 to 5 minutes. Transfer the shrimp to the bowl with the vegetables.

Add the sesame oil to the pan and cook the scallion whites, garlic, and ginger for just 30 seconds. Stir in the grated cauliflower, along with the tamari and black pepper. Cook until the cauliflower is tender, about 3 minutes. Transfer the cauliflower to the bowl with the vegetables and shrimp. Garnish with the scallion greens and serve.

Nutritional analysis per serving: Calories: 440, Fat: 19 g, Saturated Fat: 3.5 g, Cholesterol: 280 mg, Fiber: 12 g, Protein: 34 g, Carbohydrates: 39 g, Sodium: 525 mg

HOT AND SPICY SHRIMP WITH CORIANDER

Serves: 4

Prep Time:
15 minutes

Cook Time:
10 minutes

Chile peppers are graded on the Scoville scale to measure their heat. At the bottom of the scale are mild peppers such as bell peppers and pimientos. Moderate-heat peppers include ancho and poblano peppers. And for those of you who enjoy more heat, jalapeños, cayennes, and Scotch bonnets offer a nice hit of spice. For a less spicy version of this recipe, try using only one jalapeño. And remember that most of a chile pepper's heat is contained in the seeds!

- 3 tablespoons grapeseed oil
- 1 pound medium shrimp, peeled and deveined
- ½ teaspoon ground coriander
- ¼ teaspoon cayenne pepper
- sea salt
- 2 long red sweet chiles (such as Anaheim), seeded and thinly sliced
- 3 jalapeños, seeded and thinly sliced
- 3 leeks, halved lengthwise and cut crosswise into 1-inch-thick slices, white and pale green parts only
- 4 garlic cloves, thinly sliced
- 1 bunch cilantro, stems included, finely chopped, plus additional leaves for garnish

Heat 1 tablespoon of the oil in a large skillet over medium-high heat until shimmering. Sprinkle the shrimp with the coriander, cayenne, and ¼ teaspoon salt. Add to the hot oil and cook, stirring, until lightly browned and just opaque, 2 to 3 minutes. Transfer to a plate.

Heat another tablespoon of oil in the same skillet. Add the sweet chiles, jalapeños, and ¼ teaspoon salt. Cook, stirring occasionally, until crisp-tender, 1 to 2 minutes. Transfer to the plate with the shrimp.

Heat the remaining tablespoon of oil in the same skillet. Add the leeks, garlic, and a pinch of salt. Cook, stirring occasionally, until the leeks are lightly browned and crisp-tender, about 3 minutes. Add the shrimp, chiles, and chopped cilantro and mix well.

Serve garnished with cilantro leaves.

Nutritional analysis per serving: *Calories 293, Fat 12 g, Saturated Fat 1 g, Cholesterol 183 mg, Fiber 4 g, Protein 26 g, Carbohydrates 23 g, Sodium 477 mg*

BROILED SALMON WITH ALMOND-DILL SAUCE

When purchasing salmon, try to choose only wild-caught; it is less environmentally damaging than farmed salmon and much higher in healthy omega-3 fats. If you leave the skin on, you'll get even more of those healthy fats, as they are richest in the skin and just beneath it.

- 1½ cups unsweetened almond milk
- grated zest and juice of 1 lemon
- 3 garlic cloves, minced
- ½ teaspoon Dijon mustard
- pinch of ground cumin
- freshly ground black pepper
- 3 tablespoons finely chopped fresh dill, plus more for garnish
- 2 tablespoons Mayonnaise (page 299) or Vegenaise
- 2 tablespoons extra-virgin olive oil
- ¼ teaspoon ground sage
- 4 (8-ounce) boneless, skin-on wild salmon steaks
- ¼ teaspoon sea salt

Serves: 4

Prep Time: 10 minutes, plus chilling time

Cook Time: 50 minutes

Combine the almond milk, lemon zest, 1 tablespoon of the minced garlic, the mustard, cumin, and a pinch of black pepper in a 2-quart saucepan. Bring to a boil over medium heat and cook, stirring occasionally, until the liquid has reduced to about ⅓ cup, 35 to 40 minutes. Transfer the liquid to a heatproof bowl and chill in the freezer until cool, about 20 minutes (stirring after 10 minutes). Once fully chilled, whisk in the lemon juice, dill, and mayonnaise. Cover and refrigerate until serving time.

Preheat the broiler. Line a rimmed baking sheet with foil.

In a small bowl, stir together 1 tablespoon of the oil, the remaining garlic, and the sage. Set aside.

Brush the salmon steaks on both sides with the remaining 1 tablespoon oil and sprinkle with the salt. Place the steaks, skin-side up, on the lined baking sheet. Cook about 5 inches below the broiler until the outside is opaque and the skin is beginning to crisp, 4 to 6 minutes. Turn the steaks and continue to cook for another 4 minutes, then brush with the garlic mixture. Continue to cook until the salmon is still pink in the center but warm throughout, about 1 minute. Place the salmon steaks on serving plates, spoon the chilled almond–dill sauce over them, garnish with additional dill, and serve.

Nutritional analysis per serving: Calories: 454, Fat: 28 g, Saturated Fat: 4 g, Cholesterol: 127 mg, Fiber: 1 g, Protein: 46 g, Carbohydrates: 2 g, Sodium: 358 mg

ROASTED SALMON WITH GREEN BEANS

Serves: 4

Prep Time:
10 minutes

Cook Time:
10 minutes

We all need a simple "go to" salmon recipe that never lets us down, and this is it!

- 2 tablespoons plus ¼ teaspoon sea salt
- 1½ pounds green beans, trimmed
- 1 teaspoon extra-virgin olive oil
- grated zest of 1 lemon
- 4 (6-ounce) boneless, skinless wild salmon fillets
- 3 tablespoons Dijon mustard
- ½ cup finely chopped fresh dill
- 1 tablespoon grapeseed oil

Preheat the broiler. Line a rimmed baking sheet with foil.

Bring a 5-quart pot of water to a boil over high heat. Add 2 tablespoons of the salt. Cook the green beans until crisp-tender, 3 to 4 minutes. Drain the beans in a colander and rinse with cold water. Gently pat the beans dry with paper towels and transfer to a large bowl. Toss with the olive oil, lemon zest, and remaining ¼ teaspoon salt. Set aside.

Pat the salmon fillets dry with paper towels and place on the lined baking sheet. Spread an equal amount of mustard over the top of each fillet. Divide the dill among the fillets, patting it gently into the mustard. Drizzle the tops of the fillets with the grapeseed oil to prevent the herbs from browning too much.

Place the salmon under the broiler and cook until the dill is a bit frizzled and the center of the fish is tender and pink, 6 to 8 minutes. Serve with the green beans on the side.

Nutritional analysis per serving: *Calories: 335, Fat: 16 g, Saturated Fat: 2 g, Cholesterol: 94 mg, Fiber: 5 g, Protein: 37 g, Carbohydrates: 12 g, Sodium: 348 mg*

SALMON BURGERS WITH PICKLED RADISHES AND AVOCADO

Serves: 4

Prep Time:
30 minutes

Cook Time:
6 minutes

I love the zesty zing the pickled radishes provide in this recipe. Enjoy their flavor while your body is flooded with cancer-fighting isothiocyanates and antioxidants like vitamin C.

- 4 or 5 large red radishes, very thinly sliced
- 2 teaspoons fresh lemon or lime juice
- sea salt and freshly ground black pepper
- 1 pound boneless, skinless wild salmon fillets, cut into 2-inch pieces
- ¼ red onion, finely diced
- ¼ cup chopped fresh mixed herbs (such as parsley, mint, cilantro, and/or dill)
- ½ teaspoon minced fresh ginger
- ½ teaspoon ground turmeric
- ½ teaspoon ground cumin
- ½ teaspoon ground coriander
- ¼ cup sesame seeds, preferably mixed black and white
- 1 tablespoon extra-virgin olive oil
- 4 large lettuce leaves (such as romaine, green leaf, or red leaf)
- 1 avocado, pitted, peeled, and sliced, for garnish

In a small bowl, toss the radishes with 1 teaspoon of the citrus juice and ½ teaspoon salt. Set aside.

Place the salmon pieces in a food processor and pulse about 8 times to coarsely chop. Don't let the machine run and puree the fish; you want chickpea-size pieces.

Transfer the chopped fish to a bowl and fold in the onion and herbs. Add the remaining 1 teaspoon citrus juice and ½ teaspoon salt, along with the ginger, turmeric, cumin, coriander, and a pinch of black pepper and mix well.

Spread the sesame seeds on a small plate. Wet your hands, and form the salmon into 4 equal-size patties. Press the sesame seeds onto both sides of each patty and set them on a plate.

Heat the olive oil in a large cast-iron skillet or sauté pan over high heat until shimmering. Gently place the salmon burgers in the pan and cook until browned on the outside and cooked through, about 3 minutes per side.

Place one lettuce leaf on each plate and place a burger on top. Garnish the burgers with the pickled radishes and sliced avocado and serve.

Nutritional analysis per serving: *Calories: 320, Fat: 21 g, Saturated Fat: 2.5 g, Cholesterol: 60 mg, Fiber: 5 g, Protein: 25 g, Carbohydrates: 7 g, Sodium: 550 mg*

ROASTED SALMON AND ASPARAGUS WITH HERB-AVOCADO MASH

On busy evenings, I love a recipe that simplifies the cooking process, and this recipe does just that—the asparagus and salmon roast at the same time! Dinner is on the table in a jiffy.

- 1 tablespoon grapeseed oil
- 4 (6-ounce) boneless, skin-on wild salmon fillets
- 24 asparagus spears, trimmed
- 1 tablespoon extra-virgin olive oil
- sea salt and freshly ground black pepper
- 1 avocado, pitted, peeled, and mashed
- 1 tablespoon minced fresh chives
- 1 tablespoon chopped fresh mint
- 1 tablespoon chopped fresh basil
- 1 tablespoon chopped fresh cilantro or parsley
- 1 scallion, finely chopped
- ½ teaspoon fresh lemon or lime juice

Preheat the oven to 400°F.

Brush two rimmed sheet pans with the grapeseed oil. Place the salmon fillets on one sheet and the asparagus on the other sheet. Drizzle the olive oil over the salmon and asparagus, making sure to coat both well. Sprinkle both with ½ teaspoon each salt and black pepper.

Place both sheet pans in the oven and roast until the salmon is just cooked through and the asparagus just begins to wrinkle, 8 to 10 minutes. Depending on the thickness of the asparagus, you may need to leave it in for a few more minutes. Remove both pans from the oven and set aside.

In a small bowl combine the avocado with the herbs, scallion, citrus juice, and a pinch of black pepper. Mix well.

Place a salmon fillet on each plate, along with a spoonful of the mashed avocado and 6 asparagus spears. Serve.

Nutritional analysis per serving: *Calories: 404, Fat: 25 g, Saturated Fat: 4 g, Cholesterol: 94 mg, Fiber: 6 g, Protein: 37 g, Carbohydrates: 9 g, Sodium: 429 mg*

SLOW-COOKED SALMON WITH ASIAN GREENS

Serves: 4

Prep Time:
10 minutes

Cook Time:
20 minutes

Ground turmeric gives the rub for this salmon a beautiful color. Food is medicine, and this recipe certainly celebrates that with the anti-inflammatory compound curcumin in the turmeric, not to mention the anti-inflammatory fats in the salmon. This meal has all the right ingredients to transform your health.

- 1 tablespoon extra-virgin olive oil
- 1 teaspoon ground turmeric
- 1 teaspoon ground coriander
- sea salt and freshly ground black pepper
- 4 (5-ounce) boneless, skin-on wild salmon fillets
- 3 tablespoons grapeseed oil
- 2 shallots, very thinly sliced
- 1¼ pounds bok choy, thinly sliced
- 5 ounces baby spinach
- 1 teaspoon toasted sesame seeds, for garnish (optional)

Preheat the oven to 275°F. Line a rimmed baking sheet with foil.

In a small bowl, combine the olive oil, turmeric, coriander, ½ teaspoon salt, and ¼ teaspoon black pepper. Rub the mixture on the flesh of the salmon fillets (not the skin). Place the fillets, skin-side up, on the lined baking sheet. Bake until just cooked through, about 20 minutes.

Meanwhile, in a large skillet, heat the grapeseed oil over medium heat until shimmering. Add the shallots and cook, stirring frequently, until crisp and brown, about 5 minutes. Transfer with a slotted spoon to paper towels to drain. Sprinkle with a pinch of salt.

Raise the heat to medium-high and add the bok choy, ¼ teaspoon salt, and a pinch of black pepper. Cook, stirring frequently, until bright green and crisp-tender, about 4 minutes. Add the spinach and season with ¼ teaspoon each salt and black pepper. Cook, stirring, until just wilted, about 1 minute. Divide the greens among four serving plates.

Peel off and discard the salmon skins. Place the fillets on top of the greens and garnish with the crisp shallots and sesame seeds, if desired.

Nutritional analysis per serving: *Calories: 370, Fat: 23 g, Saturated Fat: 3 g, Cholesterol: 80 mg, Fiber: 4 g, Protein: 32 g, Carbohydrates: 11 g, Sodium: 430 mg*

CHIPOTLE SALMON WITH ARUGULA SALAD

Serves: 4

Prep Time:
20 minutes

Cook Time:
40 minutes

The balsamic vinegar in this recipe lends a subtle sweetness and depth to the smoky-spicy chipotle. The combination of flavors will quickly captivate your taste buds and make this a family favorite.

- 1 large head cauliflower, cored and cut into 2-inch florets
- 2 tablespoons extra-virgin olive oil
- sea salt and freshly ground black pepper
- 1 (7-ounce) can chipotle peppers in adobo sauce, peppers seeded and minced, 2 teaspoons sauce reserved
- 1 tablespoon balsamic vinegar
- 4 (4- to 6-ounce) boneless, skin-on wild salmon fillets
- 2 cups baby arugula
- ¼ cup chopped sun-dried tomatoes
- ¼ cup chopped Kalamata olives
- 2 tablespoons pine nuts
- 1 tablespoon cider vinegar
- 1½ teaspoons Dijon mustard

Preheat the oven to 450°F.

Place the cauliflower florets on a large rimmed baking sheet. Drizzle with 1 tablespoon of the olive oil and season with ¼ teaspoon salt and a pinch of black pepper. Toss to coat the cauliflower with the oil and seasonings. Roast the cauliflower, stirring once midway, until it is tender and golden, 25 to 30 minutes. Remove from the oven and reduce the temperature to 400°F.

In a small bowl, stir together the chipotle peppers, adobo sauce, and balsamic vinegar. Place the salmon fillets, skin-side down, in a baking dish. Use a spoon or a brush to coat the top of the salmon with the chipotle mixture. Bake until the salmon is cooked through, 12 to 16 minutes, depending on the thickness.

Meanwhile, in a large bowl, combine the roasted cauliflower, arugula, sun-dried tomatoes, olives, and pine nuts. In a small bowl, whisk together the remaining 1 tablespoon olive oil, the cider vinegar, mustard, and a pinch of salt. Drizzle the dressing over the salad, gently tossing to combine. Serve with the salmon.

Nutritional analysis per serving: *Calories: 416, Fat: 25 g, Saturated Fat: 3 g, Cholesterol: 65 mg, Fiber: 8 g, Protein: 30 g, Carbohydrates: 22 g, Sodium: 519 mg*

GRILLED SALMON WITH CUCUMBER SALAD

Serves: 4

Prep Time:
15 minutes

Cook Time:
10 minutes

Caraway seeds have a similar taste to licorice and fennel. If you like the flavor of rye bread, then you will enjoy the cucumber salad. I serve this meal for weekend brunch because the dill and caraway remind me of refreshing, uplifting Sunday mornings.

- ¼ cup apple cider vinegar
- 1 tablespoon caraway seeds
- 1 tablespoon yellow mustard seeds
- sea salt and freshly ground black pepper
- 2 large seedless cucumbers, thinly sliced
- 4 (6-ounce) boneless, skin-on wild salmon fillets
- 5½ ounces baby arugula
- 1 Belgian endive, thinly sliced
- ½ cup chopped fresh dill, plus more for garnish
- 1 tablespoon almond or extra-virgin olive oil
- grated zest and juice of 1 lemon

Combine the vinegar, caraway seeds, mustard seeds, ½ teaspoon salt, and a pinch of black pepper in a large bowl. Add the cucumbers and stir to coat. Let stand, stirring occasionally, while you prepare the salmon.

Heat a well-seasoned stovetop grill pan or large skillet over medium heat. Sprinkle the flesh side of the salmon fillets with ¼ teaspoon each salt and black pepper. Place the fillets, skin-side up, in the pan and cook until the flesh releases easily from the bottom, about 5 minutes. Turn and cook until the salmon is just opaque throughout, about 4 more minutes.

While the salmon cooks, toss the arugula, endive, dill, and almond oil with the cucumber mixture. Divide the salad among four plates. Top each with a salmon fillet and garnish with the lemon zest, lemon juice, and additional dill. Serve.

Nutritional analysis per serving: *Calories: 339, Fat: 16 g, Saturated Fat: 2 g, Cholesterol: 94 mg, Fiber: 3 g, Protein: 37 g, Carbohydrates: 13 g, Sodium: 525 mg*

ASIAN-SPICED SALMON CAKES

Serves: 4

Prep Time:
30 minutes

Cook Time:
5 minutes

These salmon cakes are moist and full of flavor. Double the batch and call some friends over to enjoy together!

- 2 large seedless cucumbers, halved lengthwise and thinly sliced
- 2 medium shallots, 1 thinly sliced, 1 minced
- 3 tablespoons apple cider vinegar
- 1 tablespoon plus 1 teaspoon gluten-free, low-sodium tamari
- ½ teaspoon toasted sesame oil
- sea salt
- 1 head napa cabbage, cut into 1-inch pieces
- 1¼ pounds boneless, skinless wild salmon fillets, cut into 1-inch pieces
- 3 ounces snow peas, trimmed and thinly sliced
- 3 tablespoons Mayonnaise (page 299) or Vegenaise
- 1 tablespoon five-spice powder
- 1 tablespoon grapeseed oil

In a medium bowl, toss the cucumber and sliced shallot with 2 tablespoons of the vinegar, 1 teaspoon of the tamari, the sesame oil, and a pinch of salt. Let stand while you prepare the salmon cakes.

Pulse the napa cabbage in a food processor until very finely chopped. Transfer to a colander and toss with ¼ teaspoon salt; let stand.

Combine the minced shallot and remaining 1 tablespoon vinegar in a large bowl. Pulse three-quarters of the salmon in the food processor until finely ground. Transfer to the bowl with the shallot. Pulse the remaining salmon until just coarsely chopped. Transfer to the bowl, along with the snow peas, mayonnaise, remaining 1 tablespoon tamari, five-spice powder, and ¼ teaspoon salt. Squeeze as much liquid as possible out of the cabbage with your hands. Add the cabbage to the salmon mixture. Mix well with your hands and shape into 4 equal-size patties.

Heat the grapeseed oil in a large nonstick skillet over medium-high heat until shimmering. Add the patties and cook until browned and just cooked through, 2 to 3 minutes per side. Serve with the cucumber salad on the side.

Nutritional analysis per serving: *Calories: 311, Fat: 15 g, Saturated Fat: 2 g, Cholesterol: 80 mg, Fiber: 2 g, Protein: 31 g, Carbohydrates: 12 g, Sodium: 577 mg*

WHOLE SNAPPER STUFFED WITH SCALLION AND GINGER

Serves: 4

Prep Time:
15 minutes

Cook Time:
40 minutes

Cooking a whole fish is not as intimidating as it sounds, and the result is a sweet and delicate fish that easily flakes with the touch of your fork. Look for fish with brightly colored fins, clear eyes, and a sweet smell. Avoid purchasing anything that smells, well, fishy! Ask the fishmonger to scale, gut, and butterfly the fish for you.

- 1 head napa cabbage, cut into 3-inch pieces
- 5 large scallions, cut into 2-inch pieces
- 1 (4-inch) piece ginger, peeled and thinly sliced
- 2 tablespoons toasted sesame oil
- 1 teaspoon sea salt
- 1 teaspoon freshly ground black pepper
- 1 (2½-pound) whole wild red snapper, scaled, gutted, and butterflied
- 3 tablespoons gluten-free, low-sodium tamari

Preheat the oven to 425°F. Tear off a 4-foot length of foil and a 3-foot length of parchment paper. Place the foil on a large rimmed baking sheet, then lay the parchment paper on top.

In a large bowl, combine the cabbage, two-thirds of the scallions and ginger, 1 tablespoon of the sesame oil, and ½ teaspoon each of the salt and black pepper. Mix to coat evenly. Spread the cabbage in an even layer on the parchment paper to form a bed for the fish.

Place the fish on top of the cabbage and sprinkle the outside and cavity with the remaining ½ teaspoon each salt and black pepper. Stuff the remaining scallions and ginger slices in the cavity of the fish.

Combine the tamari with ¼ cup of water and pour over the fish. Bring up the sides of the parchment and fold it over the fish to encase it, then bring together the foil edges and crimp tightly to seal.

Bake for 40 minutes. Carefully open the packet and drizzle the remaining 1 tablespoon sesame oil over the fish. Serve the fish (discarding bones and fins) with the cabbage.

Nutritional analysis per serving: *Calories: 230, Fat: 9 g, Saturated Fat: 1.5 g, Cholesterol: 40 mg, Fiber: 3 g, Protein: 28 g, Carbohydrates: 11 g, Sodium: 540 mg*

STEAMED RED SNAPPER AND VEGETABLES EN PAPILLOTE

Serves: 4

Prep Time:
35 minutes

Cook Time:
18 minutes

En papillote literally means "in paper." This culinary trick produces a light dish yet doesn't skimp on flavor or texture. Cooking in paper allows you to preserve the crisp nature of lightly cooked vegetables while maintaining the firm flesh of the snapper.

- 2 (5.4-ounce) cans chilled unsweetened coconut cream, liquid poured off, solid cream reserved
- 1 celery root, peeled and finely chopped
- 1 cup cauliflower florets, broken into small pieces
- 2 shallots, thinly sliced
- grated zest and juice of 2 limes
- ½ teaspoon curry powder
- ½ teaspoon sea salt
- 4 (4-ounce) skinless red snapper fillets
- 2 jalapeños, seeded and thinly sliced

Preheat the oven to 400°F. Place two large rimmed baking sheets in the oven to preheat them.

Set aside 2 tablespoons of the coconut cream. In a medium bowl, combine the remaining coconut cream, celery root, cauliflower, shallots, lime zest and juice, curry powder, and salt. Set aside.

Fold four 16 x 24–inch rectangles of parchment paper in half (forming 16 x 12–inch rectangles), cut each into a half-heart shape, and open (check out an online video tutorial if necessary). Divide the celery root mixture among the parchment hearts, forming a bed on one side of each heart. Place a red snapper fillet on top of each bed of celery root. Brush each fillet with the reserved coconut cream. Top the fillets with the jalapeño slices.

To seal the packets, fold the parchment flap over the snapper; make small overlapping folds along the edges to seal.

Using a large spatula, place the packets on the preheated baking sheets. Bake, rotating the baking sheets midway, until the packets have puffed,

15 to 18 minutes; the fish will be cooked through by then. Transfer each packet to a serving plate. Serve immediately, taking care to open the packets slowly to avoid being burned by the steam.

Nutritional analysis per serving: *Calories: 360, Fat: 17 g, Saturated Fat: 14 g, Cholesterol: 40 mg, Fiber: 6 g, Protein: 29 g, Carbohydrates: 28 g, Sodium: 480 mg*

Bok Choy Stir-Fry with Black Cod

Serves: 4

Prep Time:
20 minutes

Cook Time:
16 minutes

This dish celebrates the buttery flavor that oily fish offer. Look for bluefish, mackerel, Arctic char, or steelhead trout if you can't find black cod. Be sure to pick out any pin bones from the cod that the fishmonger may have missed. Serve with a side of Cauliflower "Rice" (page 264).

- 4 tablespoons grapeseed oil
- 4 (4-ounce) boneless, skin-on black cod (or other oily fish) fillets
- sea salt
- 3 garlic cloves, minced
- 1 (1-inch) piece ginger, peeled and minced
- 8 ounces shiitake mushrooms, stems removed, caps cut into ¼-inch-thick slices
- 4 scallions, cut on the bias into 1-inch pieces
- 1 tablespoon gluten-free, low-sodium tamari
- 1 red bell pepper, seeded and thinly sliced
- 1 pound baby bok choy, trimmed, halved lengthwise if large

Heat a well-seasoned stovetop grill pan or large skillet over medium-high heat. Rub 1 tablespoon of the oil all over the fish and sprinkle the flesh side with ¼ teaspoon salt. Place the fillets, skin-side up, in the hot pan. Cook until the flesh releases easily from the pan, about 5 minutes. Carefully turn each piece over and cook just until opaque throughout, about 3 minutes. Transfer to a plate.

While the fish cooks, heat 1 tablespoon of the oil in a large skillet over medium-high heat until shimmering. Add half of the garlic and ginger and cook, stirring, for 5 seconds. Add the mushrooms, scallions, 1½ tablespoons of water, and a pinch of salt. Cook, stirring occasionally, until the mushrooms are lightly browned and tender, about 5 minutes. Stir in the tamari, then transfer the mixture to a bowl.

Heat the remaining 2 tablespoons oil in the same skillet. Add the remaining garlic and ginger and cook, stirring, for 5 seconds. Add the bell pepper, bok choy, 1½ tablespoons of water, and ¼ teaspoon salt.

Cook, stirring, just until the vegetables are crisp-tender, about 3 minutes. Return the mushroom mixture to the skillet and fold gently to mix. Divide among four serving plates and top with the grilled fish. Serve.

Nutritional analysis per serving: *Calories: 367, Fat: 28 g, Saturated Fat: 5 g, Cholesterol: 56 mg, Fiber: 4 g, Protein: 19 g, Carbohydrates: 10 g, Sodium: 489 mg*

MISO-MARINATED COD WITH FRESH BASIL AND BOK CHOY

Serves: 4

Prep Time:
20 minutes

Cook Time:
10 minutes

This is a great last-minute dish, and even better if you have the time to allow the fish to marinate. Start the bok choy when you're ready to cook the fish.

- 2 tablespoons plus ¼ teaspoon sea salt
- 1 large head bok choy (about 1½ pounds), stems and leaves separated and cut into ½-inch-thick pieces
- 1 teaspoon toasted sesame oil
- ¼ cup gluten-free, low-sodium white miso
- 3 tablespoons apple cider vinegar
- 4 garlic cloves, minced
- ¼ teaspoon cayenne pepper
- 4 (6-ounce) skinless wild-caught cod fillets
- ¼ cup chopped fresh basil, for garnish
- 2 teaspoons toasted sesame seeds, for garnish
- ¼ teaspoon crushed red pepper flakes, for garnish

Preheat the broiler. Line a rimmed baking sheet with foil.

Bring a 5-quart pot of water to a boil over high heat. Add 2 tablespoons of the salt. Cook the bok choy stems until they start to become translucent, 2 to 3 minutes. Then, add the leaves and continue to cook until the leaves are tender, another 1 to 2 minutes. Drain the bok choy in a colander, gently pat dry with paper towels, and transfer to a medium bowl. Toss with the sesame oil and the remaining ¼ teaspoon salt. Set aside.

In a small bowl, whisk together the miso, vinegar, garlic, and cayenne. Pat the fish dry with paper towels and place on the lined baking sheet. Spread the miso mixture over the top of each fish fillet.

Place the fish under the broiler until the top is a bit dry and the fish is cooked through, 6 to 8 minutes. Garnish the fish with basil, sesame seeds, and red pepper flakes. Serve with bok choy on the side.

Nutritional analysis per serving: *Calories 221, Fat 4 g, Saturated Fat 1 g, Cholesterol 73 mg, Fiber 2 g, Protein 34 g, Carbohydrates 13 g, Sodium 619 mg*

Cod Cakes with Miso Eggplant

Serves: 4

Prep Time: 20 minutes, plus chilling time

Cook Time: 40 minutes

This is one dish you won't want to skip—especially if you love the refreshing, zesty flavor of lime that is beautifully infused in each bite of cod. The miso eggplant is sure to impress, with its unforgettable umami, or savory, flavor.

- 4½ tablespoons extra-virgin olive oil
- 1 pound skinless wild-caught cod fillets
- ¼ teaspoon sea salt
- 3 tablespoons gluten-free, low-sodium white miso
- 1 tablespoon rice wine vinegar
- 1 garlic clove, minced
- 2 small eggplants, cut crosswise into ½-inch slices
- ½ teaspoon sesame seeds (optional)
- 2 large omega-3 eggs
- 2 scallions, thinly sliced, plus more for garnish
- ½ teaspoon grated fresh lime zest
- 2 tablespoons fresh lime juice
- 1 cup coconut flour
- ½ cup Mayonnaise (page 299) or Vegenaise
- 2 teaspoons wasabi paste

Preheat the oven to 400°F.

Brush a rimmed baking sheet with ½ tablespoon of the oil. Place the cod fillets on the sheet; season with a pinch of salt. Roast until cooked through, 6 to 8 minutes. Transfer the fillets to a plate and refrigerate to cool completely, 10 to 15 minutes; if any moisture accumulates after cooling, pat dry with paper towels. With a fork, flake the fish into small pieces.

Preheat the broiler. Line a large rimmed baking sheet with foil.

In a small bowl, combine the miso, vinegar, and garlic. Set aside.

Brush both sides of the eggplant slices with 2 tablespoons of the oil and arrange them on the lined baking sheet. Place them 2 to 3 inches

171

under the broiler and broil until golden brown and beginning to soften, 10 to 12 minutes, flipping the slices halfway through cooking.

Spread the miso mixture evenly over each slice of eggplant. Return to the broiler and cook until the miso is bubbling and the eggplant is tender, 8 to 10 minutes. If the miso begins to get too dark, cover the eggplant with foil and continue to cook. Sprinkle with sesame seeds, if desired. Set aside.

In a large bowl, combine the eggs, scallions, lime zest and juice, and remaining salt. Fold in the fish and ¼ cup of the coconut flour. Place the remaining coconut flour on a plate. Form 8 equal-size cakes, using about ¼ cup of fish mixture for each. Dredge the cakes in the flour, gently pressing to adhere.

In a small bowl, whisk together the mayonnaise and wasabi paste and set aside.

Warm the remaining 2 tablespoons oil in a 10-inch skillet over medium heat until shimmering. Place 4 cakes in the skillet and cook until golden brown, 2 to 4 minutes per side. Repeat with the remaining cakes. Serve with the eggplant and wasabi mayo on the side.

Nutritional analysis per serving: Calories: 522, Fat: 29 g, Saturated Fat: 8 g, Cholesterol: 168 mg, Fiber: 14 g, Protein: 30 g, Carbohydrates: 37 g, Sodium: 624 mg

Chicken and Turkey

BRAISED CHICKEN WITH ONIONS AND PEPPERS

Serves: 4

Prep Time:
25 minutes

Cook Time:
1 hour and
15 minutes

The sauce from the chicken, vegetables, and herbs will make you return to this recipe time and time again.

- 1 tablespoon coconut oil
- 1¼ pounds boneless, skinless chicken thighs
- ½ teaspoon sea salt
- ½ teaspoon freshly ground black pepper
- 4 medium yellow onions, halved and thinly sliced
- 2 green bell peppers, seeded and thinly sliced
- 4 red bell peppers, seeded and thinly sliced
- 3 garlic cloves, thinly sliced
- ⅓ cup apple cider vinegar
- ⅓ cup low-sodium chicken stock
- ½ teaspoon dried thyme
- 4 to 6 cups arugula or spinach

In a large Dutch oven, warm the oil over medium-high heat until shimmering. Season the chicken thighs with ¼ teaspoon each salt and black pepper. Brown the chicken thighs, 4 to 5 minutes on each side. Transfer the chicken to a plate.

Add the onions to the skillet and cook, stirring occasionally, until softened, about 10 minutes. Stir in the bell peppers and cook for another 10 minutes, stirring occasionally. Add the garlic and continue cooking for 1 minute, stirring constantly.

Add the vinegar, chicken stock, thyme, and remaining ¼ teaspoon each salt and black pepper. Stir well, scraping up the brown bits from the bottom of the pan.

Using a wooden spoon, make four little vegetable "nests" and lay a chicken thigh in each. Bring the liquid to a boil, then reduce to a simmer over low heat. Cover and cook until the chicken is tender and cooked through, about 35 minutes. Check occasionally to make sure the liquid is at a simmer.

Use a slotted spoon to transfer the chicken and vegetables to a platter. Bring the remaining liquid to a boil over high heat. Cook until most of the liquid has evaporated and only a few tablespoons of thickened sauce are left, 5 to 10 minutes.

Divide the greens among four plates. Top with the vegetables and chicken, drizzle sauce over both, and serve.

Nutritional analysis per serving: *Calories: 320, Fat: 10 g, Saturated Fat: 4.5 g, Cholesterol: 135 mg, Fiber: 7 g, Protein: 30 g, Carbohydrates: 27 g, Sodium: 450 mg*

MOROCCAN CHICKEN AND VEGETABLE STEW

This is a vegetable-loaded version of the classic Moroccan stew called a *tagine*. Tagines are usually made with lamb or chicken, with lots of warm spices, ginger, and dried fruit.

- ¼ cup extra-virgin olive oil
- 2 yellow onions, diced
- 6 garlic cloves, minced
- 1 tablespoon minced fresh ginger
- 1 teaspoon sea salt
- 2 teaspoons ground turmeric
- 2 teaspoons ground cumin
- 2 teaspoons ground coriander
- 2 teaspoons ground ginger
- ½ teaspoon ground cinnamon
- pinch of cayenne pepper
- 4 boneless, skinless chicken thighs, cut into 2-inch pieces
- ½ head cauliflower, cored and cut into 2-inch florets
- 8 to 10 button mushrooms, trimmed and quartered
- 1 eggplant, peeled and cut into 1-inch dice
- 1 large red bell pepper, seeded and cut into 1-inch pieces
- 1 zucchini, sliced into ½-inch-thick rounds
- 2 cups low-sodium chicken or vegetable stock
- 10 grape tomatoes, halved
- ¼ cup sliced green olives
- ¼ cup sliced almonds
- chopped fresh cilantro, for garnish

In a Dutch oven or heavy stockpot, heat the olive oil over medium-low heat. Add the onions, garlic, and fresh ginger and sauté gently until the onions begin to caramelize, 10 to 15 minutes.

Turn the heat to low, and add ¾ teaspoon of the salt and all of the dried spices. Sauté the spices and onions until fragrant, about 2 minutes.

Sprinkle the chicken with the remaining ¼ teaspoon salt. Turn the heat to medium, add the chicken to the pan, and sauté for 3 minutes, stirring to coat well with the spices.

Add the cauliflower and mushrooms and sauté until they begin to wilt and soften, about 5 minutes.

Add the eggplant, bell pepper, and zucchini and sauté until they soften, about 5 minutes.

Add the chicken stock and bring to a simmer. It will look as though there isn't enough liquid, but as the vegetables cook down they will release a lot of water.

Simmer the stew gently, stirring occasionally, until all of the vegetables are tender and the liquid is thickened and reduced, 15 to 20 minutes.

Stir in the tomatoes and cook for 1 more minute. Stir in the olives and almonds. Serve garnished with cilantro.

Nutritional analysis per serving: Calories: 410, Fat: 23 g, Saturated Fat: 3.5 g, Cholesterol: 80 mg, Fiber: 12 g, Protein: 23 g, Carbohydrates: 32 g, Sodium: 551 mg

BALSAMIC CHICKEN WITH SAUTÉED BRUSSELS SPROUTS

Serves: 4

Prep Time:
20 minutes

Cook Time:
35 minutes

This dish can be made with any combination of chicken drumsticks, leg–thigh pieces, or bone-in breast halves. Preshredded Brussels sprouts can be purchased in the produce section of many supermarkets. If you can't find them, thinly slice trimmed sprouts, or substitute thinly sliced green cabbage.

- 4 (6-ounce) bone-in, skin-on chicken thighs
- sea salt and freshly ground black pepper
- 2 tablespoons extra-virgin olive oil
- 1 medium yellow onion, finely diced
- 3 garlic cloves, minced
- 1 medium celery rib, diced
- ½ fennel bulb, diced
- 1 small carrot, peeled and diced
- 1 cup sliced button or cremini mushrooms
- 3 tablespoons balsamic vinegar
- 1 bay leaf
- 1 large thyme sprig or ¼ teaspoon dried thyme
- 1 cup low-sodium chicken stock
- 1 pound Brussels sprouts, shredded

Pat the chicken dry with paper towels and sprinkle with ½ teaspoon salt and a pinch of black pepper. Heat 1 tablespoon of the olive oil in a large sauté pan over medium–high heat until shimmering. When the oil is hot, add the chicken, skin-side down, and sauté until the skin is golden brown, 2 to 3 minutes. Turn the thighs and sauté for another 2 minutes. Remove the chicken from the pan and set aside.

Add the onion, garlic, celery, and fennel and sauté until the vegetables are soft and beginning to brown, 3 to 5 minutes. Add the carrot and mushrooms and continue to sauté until the mushrooms are very soft and wilted, 2 to 3 minutes.

Return the chicken to the pan. Drizzle the balsamic vinegar over the chicken, add the bay leaf and thyme, and then add the chicken stock.

177

Bring to a simmer, then partially cover the pan and turn the heat to low. Simmer for 15 minutes.

Remove the chicken from the pan and keep it warm. Turn the heat up to medium-high and cook until the sauce has thickened and reduced in volume by half, about 5 minutes more. Return the chicken to the pan, spoon the sauce over the chicken, turn off the heat, and cover the pan.

In another sauté pan, heat the remaining 1 tablespoon olive oil over medium heat until shimmering. Add the Brussels sprouts, season with ½ teaspoon salt, and sauté until very soft, wilted, and beginning to brown, about 10 to 12 minutes. Divide the sprouts among four plates. Discard the bay leaf and thyme sprig (if using) and serve the chicken, vegetables, and sauce over the sautéed sprouts.

Nutritional analysis per serving: *Calories: 340, Fat: 15 g, Saturated Fat: 3 g, Cholesterol: 170 mg, Fiber: 4 g, Protein: 38 g, Carbohydrates: 15 g, Sodium: 568 mg*

FORTY-CLOVE BAKED CHICKEN WITH SWISS CHARD

Serves: 6

Prep Time:
20 minutes

Cook Time:
50 minutes

Don't be alarmed by the amount of garlic called for in this classic recipe; the flavor becomes very mellow and sweet after cooking. This dish tastes great with Arugula and Fennel Salad (page 252).

- 2 tablespoons extra-virgin olive oil
- 8 boneless, skinless chicken thighs
- sea salt and freshly ground black pepper
- ½ teaspoon freshly grated nutmeg
- 40 garlic cloves (from about 4 heads), peeled (see Note)
- ½ cup low-sodium chicken stock
- 1 bunch Swiss chard, stems thinly sliced and leaves roughly chopped
- 6 parsley sprigs, plus additional chopped leaves for garnish
- 6 tarragon sprigs, plus additional chopped leaves for garnish

Preheat the oven to 375°F.

Heat 1 tablespoon of the oil in a large Dutch oven over medium-high heat. Sprinkle the chicken with 1 teaspoon salt and ¼ teaspoon black pepper. Add the chicken to the Dutch oven and cook until browned on both sides, about 8 minutes total. Transfer to a plate and sprinkle with the nutmeg.

Add the garlic cloves to the Dutch oven. Cook until just golden, about 30 seconds, stirring constantly to avoid burning the garlic. Add the stock and bring to a boil, stirring and scraping up the browned bits. Return the chicken thighs and their accumulated juices to the Dutch oven and nestle them in the garlic. Top with the Swiss chard stems, parsley sprigs, tarragon sprigs, and ¼ teaspoon salt.

Cover and bake until the garlic is tender and emits a sweet aroma and the chicken is cooked through, about 35 minutes.

Discard the parsley and tarragon sprigs. Using tongs, transfer the chicken to a serving platter. Add the Swiss chard leaves, the remaining 1 tablespoon oil, and a pinch each of salt and black pepper to the Dutch oven. Set over medium heat and stir gently until the chard is just wilted and the garlic cloves have melted into a sauce, about 2 minutes. Spoon the garlicky Swiss chard mixture around the chicken and garnish with chopped parsley and tarragon. Serve.

Note: To peel lots of garlic quickly, separate the cloves from the head and put them in a metal mixing bowl. Place another bowl upside-down on top, hold the edges together, and shake vigorously so that the cloves bang against the insides of both bowls. This is a fun activity for kids—and it's much faster and easier than peeling cloves individually.

Nutritional analysis per serving: *Calories: 220, Fat: 10 g, Saturated Fat: 2 g, Cholesterol: 110 mg, Fiber: 1 g, Protein: 24 g, Carbohydrates: 9 g, Sodium: 523 mg*

GRILLED CHICKEN WITH BASIL PESTO

One of the best-kept secrets among cooks is how to prepare a moist and tasty boneless, skinless chicken breast: Simply stuff it with herbs and aromatics to enhance the flavor of the meat and give your dish personality and flair.

- ¼ cup pine nuts
- 2 garlic cloves, halved
- 2 cups tightly packed fresh basil leaves
- 6 tablespoons extra-virgin olive oil
- 2 tablespoons fresh lemon juice
- 1 teaspoon sea salt
- 6 (4-ounce) boneless, skinless chicken breasts
- 1 eggplant, sliced into ½-inch-thick rounds
- 10 ounces baby spinach

Serves: 6

Prep Time: 15 minutes

Cook Time: 45 minutes

In a food processor, pulse together the pine nuts, garlic, basil, 2 tablespoons of the olive oil, the lemon juice, and ¼ teaspoon of the salt until just combined. Transfer the pesto to a bowl.

Working with one chicken breast at a time, hold your knife horizontally and cut the breast almost in half through the middle—stop cutting about ½ inch before you reach the other edge to leave a "hinge." Then you can open up the breast like a book. Repeat with the remaining breasts. Sprinkle the chicken all over with ¼ teaspoon of the salt.

Spread the surface of each chicken breast with an equal amount of the basil pesto. Close the chicken breasts back up and brush the outsides with a little oil.

Heat a well-seasoned stovetop grill pan over medium-high heat. Cook the chicken breasts until golden brown on the outside and no longer pink in the center, 5 to 7 minutes on each side. Remove from the heat and, once cool enough to handle, slice the chicken crosswise into strips.

Meanwhile, preheat the broiler. Place the eggplant slices on a baking sheet. Brush both sides of the eggplant with the remaining oil and sprinkle with the remaining ½ teaspoon salt. Broil until browned and tender, 10 to 15 minutes on each side.

Place the spinach on a serving platter. Transfer the eggplant to the platter, top with the sliced chicken, and serve.

Nutritional analysis per serving: Calories: 460, Fat: 31 g, Saturated Fat: 4.5 g, Cholesterol: 95 mg, Fiber: 5 g, Protein: 35 g, Carbohydrates: 12 g, Sodium: 520 mg

CHICKEN WITH OVEN-ROASTED TOMATOES

I love making a sauce that highlights the fresh, bright flavor of vegetables, roasted to bring out their deeper complexities. When you cook with real, whole foods, you have the opportunity to enjoy the unique taste each ingredient contributes to the overall flavor of the dish. This recipe celebrates real food for all of its beauty, flavor, and health benefits.

- 1 yellow bell pepper, seeded and thinly sliced
- 1 orange bell pepper, seeded and thinly sliced
- 1 pint grape tomatoes, halved
- 1 shallot, minced
- 4 garlic cloves, thinly sliced
- 2 tablespoons extra-virgin olive oil
- sea salt and freshly ground black pepper
- 1 pound boneless, skinless chicken breasts, cut into bite-size pieces
- 2 tablespoons fresh lemon juice
- ¾ teaspoon smoked paprika
- ¼ cup thinly sliced green olives
- ¼ cup finely chopped fresh parsley

Preheat the oven to 450°F.

Toss the bell peppers, tomatoes, shallot, and garlic with the olive oil on a rimmed baking sheet. Season with a pinch each of salt and black pepper. Roast until the peppers are just tender and the tomatoes start to collapse, about 20 minutes.

Meanwhile, in a medium bowl, toss the chicken with 1 tablespoon of the lemon juice and the paprika. Season with a pinch each of salt and black pepper. Scatter the chicken on top of the roasted tomato mixture and roast until the chicken is just cooked through, about 10 minutes.

Add the olives, parsley, and remaining 1 tablespoon lemon juice and toss to combine. Season with a pinch each of salt and black pepper and serve.

Nutritional analysis per serving: *Calories 208, Fat 8 g, Saturated Fat 1 g, Cholesterol 73 mg, Fiber 3 g, Protein 26 g, Carbohydrates 9 g, Sodium 339 mg*

Pan-Roasted Chicken with Wild Mushroom Ragout

Serves: 4

Prep Time:
20 minutes

Cook Time:
40 minutes

One trick to cooking moist chicken breasts is to use bone-in, skin-on breasts. Here, the delicious browned bits left in the pan after sautéing the chicken are used to flavor the accompanying mushroom ragout.

- 4 (6-ounce) bone-in, skin-on chicken breasts
- sea salt and freshly ground black pepper
- 4 tablespoons extra-virgin olive oil
- 1 large garlic clove, minced
- 1 pound mixed mushrooms (such as button, cremini, shiitake, and/or oyster), trimmed and thinly sliced
- 1 teaspoon fresh lemon juice
- 1 cup low-sodium chicken stock
- 4 ounces baby arugula or mixed mesclun greens
- 1 tablespoon minced fresh chives or parsley, for garnish

Preheat the oven to 400°F.

Pat the chicken dry with paper towels and season with ½ teaspoon salt and a pinch of black pepper. Heat 1 tablespoon of the olive oil in a large oven-safe sauté pan over high heat until shimmering. Add the chicken, skin-side down, and cook until the skin is golden and releases from the pan, 2 to 3 minutes. Turn the chicken over and transfer the pan to the oven. Cook for 15 to 20 minutes, depending on size. The chicken is done when it feels firm to the touch and the internal temperature is 165°F. Transfer the chicken to a small rack set over a plate or sheet pan to catch any juices; do not wash out the pan.

Meanwhile, in a large sauté pan, heat 2 tablespoons of the olive oil over medium heat until shimmering. Add the garlic and cook for 30 seconds. Add the mushrooms and ¼ teaspoon salt and cook, stirring occasionally, until the mushrooms are very soft and beginning to brown, 8 to 10 minutes.

Sprinkle ½ teaspoon of the lemon juice over the mushrooms and add the chicken stock. Simmer until the stock reduces by half and the ragout is thickened, 5 to 7 minutes.

Transfer the mushroom ragout to the pan used to cook the chicken. Add the juices that have collected under the chicken and place the pan over low heat. Stir to release the browned chicken bits from the pan into the mushrooms, then remove from the heat.

Cut the chicken off the bone and into slices. Toss the arugula with the remaining 1 tablespoon olive oil and ½ teaspoon lemon juice. Distribute the arugula among four dinner plates and arrange the chicken slices on top. Spoon the mushroom ragout over the chicken and serve, garnished with the fresh herbs.

Nutritional analysis per serving: *Calories: 280, Fat: 18 g, Saturated Fat: 3 g, Cholesterol: 75 mg, Fiber: 1 g, Protein: 28 g, Carbohydrates: 4 g, Sodium: 490 mg*

POACHED CHICKEN WITH COLESLAW, ALMONDS, AND PEPITAS

Serves: 4

Prep Time:
15 minutes

Cook Time:
20 minutes

Celery seed is that unique flavor in coleslaw that we all love but can't put our finger on. Don't skip this ingredient because it makes the dish.

- ½ cup Mayonnaise (page 299) or Vegenaise
- 1 tablespoon Dijon mustard
- 1 tablespoon apple cider vinegar
- 1 tablespoon fresh lemon juice
- 6 garlic cloves, 3 minced and 3 halved
- ¼ teaspoon sea salt
- 1 small green cabbage, finely shredded
- 2 medium carrots, peeled and coarsely grated
- 1 small yellow onion, finely diced
- ¼ teaspoon celery seeds
- 4 (6-ounce) boneless, skinless chicken breasts
- ¼ cup slivered almonds
- ¼ cup pepitas

In a small bowl, whisk together the mayonnaise, mustard, vinegar, lemon juice, minced garlic, and salt.

In a large bowl, combine the cabbage, carrots, onion, and celery seeds. Add the dressing and toss to coat thoroughly. Cover and refrigerate until ready to serve.

Put the chicken and the halved garlic cloves in a large saucepan. Fill it almost to the top with cold water and bring to a boil over medium-high heat. Reduce the heat to a simmer and cook until the chicken is no longer pink in the center, 10 to 12 minutes or until the internal temperature reaches 165°F. Discard the garlic and transfer the chicken to a cutting board.

While the chicken is cooking, toast the almonds and pepitas in a small skillet over medium heat, stirring frequently, until they just begin to brown, 2 to 4 minutes.

Slice the chicken; serve with the slaw, and garnish with toasted almonds and pepitas.

Nutritional analysis per serving: *Calories: 468, Fat: 19 g, Saturated Fat: 3 g, Cholesterol: 116 mg, Fiber: 9 g, Protein: 44 g, Carbohydrates: 30 g, Sodium: 501 mg*

POMEGRANATE CHICKEN

Serves: 4

Prep Time:
20 minutes

Cook Time:
5 minutes

Ras el hanout is a prized Moroccan spice blend that really ties together the Middle Eastern flavors of this dish. It's available at many large supermarkets and specialty shops, or you can try mixing up your own with the recipe on page 300.

- ¼ cup fresh lemon juice
- ¼ cup tahini
- 1 garlic clove, halved
- sea salt
- 1 pound thin-cut chicken cutlets
- grated zest of 1 lemon
- 2 teaspoons ground sumac (or grated zest of another lemon)
- 2 teaspoons Ras el Hanout (page 300)
- 1 bunch chicory or 1 head escarole, chopped
- 1 head radicchio, cut in quarters, cored, and thinly sliced
- ½ cup pomegranate seeds
- ¼ cup chopped toasted walnuts
- chopped fresh parsley, cilantro, and/or mint, for garnish

Combine the lemon juice, tahini, garlic, ¼ cup of water, and a pinch of salt in a blender. Blend until smooth, 1 to 2 minutes.

Sprinkle the chicken with the lemon zest, sumac, ras el hanout, and ½ teaspoon salt. Heat a well-seasoned stovetop grill pan over medium-high heat. Add the chicken and cook, turning once, until cooked through, 3 to 4 minutes total. Transfer to a cutting board.

Toss the chicory, radicchio, and pomegranate seeds with the tahini dressing and divide among four serving plates. Slice the chicken into strips and arrange on top of the greens. Sprinkle with the walnuts and herbs and serve.

Nutritional analysis per serving: *Calories 341, Fat 17 g, Saturated Fat 2 g, Cholesterol 73 mg, Fiber 8 g, Protein 32 g, Carbohydrates 20 g, Sodium 500 mg*

CHICKEN PROVENÇAL WITH ZUCCHINI AND PEPPERS

Serves: 4

Prep Time: 15 minutes

Cook Time: 35 minutes

The term *Provençal* refers to food prepared in the style of the French region of Provence, where a fresh, whole-foods culinary approach celebrates the region's tomatoes, onions, olives, and garlic. While some people are intimidated by French cooking, even a novice chef will be able to cook this wholesome dish, which tastes as fantastic as it looks.

- 8 bone-in, skinless chicken drumsticks and/or thighs
- sea salt and freshly ground black pepper
- 1 tablespoon extra-virgin olive oil
- 1 large yellow onion, diced
- 1 celery rib, diced
- 1 small carrot, peeled and diced
- 8 garlic cloves, halved
- 2 teaspoons tomato paste
- 1 bay leaf
- 1 thyme sprig or ½ teaspoon dried thyme
- 1 small zucchini, cut into ¼-inch-thick rounds
- 1 small red bell pepper, seeded and cut into ¼-inch-thick strips
- 2 cups low-sodium chicken stock
- 2 tablespoons apple cider vinegar
- 2 tablespoons chopped fresh parsley, for garnish
- 2 teaspoons minced fresh oregano, for garnish (optional)

Pat the chicken dry and season with ¼ teaspoon salt and a pinch of black pepper. In a large sauté pan or cast-iron skillet, heat the olive oil over medium heat until shimmering. Add the chicken and cook until the pieces are browned all over, about 1 minute per side. Transfer the chicken to a plate.

Add the onion, celery, carrot, and garlic to the pan and sauté until the vegetables are soft and golden brown, 5 to 7 minutes. Stir in the tomato paste and cook for 1 minute. Add the bay leaf, thyme, zucchini, and bell pepper and cook for another 2 minutes.

Return the chicken to the pan. Add the chicken stock, vinegar, and ¼ teaspoon salt and bring to a simmer. Reduce the heat to low, cover the pan, and braise the chicken for 10 minutes.

Transfer the chicken to a plate and set aside. Increase the heat and simmer the sauce and vegetables until the sauce is reduced by half and the vegetables are very tender, about 10 minutes. Discard the bay leaf and thyme sprig (if using). Return the chicken to the pan and coat it with the vegetables and sauce.

Transfer the stew to a serving platter, sprinkle with the parsley and oregano (if desired), and serve.

Nutritional analysis per serving: *Calories: 260, Fat: 10 g, Saturated Fat: 2 g, Cholesterol: 145 mg, Fiber: 2 g, Protein: 30 g, Carbohydrates: 11 g, Sodium: 510 mg*

RATATOUILLE WITH ROASTED CHICKEN

Serves: 8

Prep Time:
30 minutes

Cook Time:
1 hour

Ratatouille is a summer vegetable stew from the south of France. Traditionally made with eggplant, bell peppers, zucchini, tomatoes, and basil, it can be served as a side dish or as a delicious base for roasted or grilled meats or fish. It's also wonderful at brunch, topped with poached eggs.

- 1 (3-pound) whole chicken
- sea salt and freshly ground black pepper
- juice of ½ lemon
- 2 bay leaves
- 2 tablespoons extra-virgin olive oil
- 4 garlic cloves, minced
- 1 small eggplant, cut into 1-inch pieces
- 1 small zucchini, cut into 1-inch pieces
- 1 small yellow summer squash, cut into 1-inch pieces
- 1 red, orange, or yellow bell pepper, seeded and cut into 1-inch pieces
- 1 tablespoon tomato paste
- 1 cup canned crushed tomatoes or chopped fresh tomatoes with their juices
- 2 tablespoons chopped fresh basil, plus more for garnish

Preheat the oven to 400°F.

Pat the chicken dry with paper towels, then place, breast-side up, in a roasting pan or baking dish. Sprinkle the chicken all over with ½ teaspoon salt and a pinch of black pepper, and squeeze the lemon juice all over the chicken. Place the squeezed lemon half and the bay leaves in the chicken cavity. Tie the legs together with kitchen twine, brush with oil, and roast the chicken, basting throughout, until an instant-read thermometer inserted in the thickest part of the thigh reads 165°F, 50 to 55 minutes. Remove the chicken from the oven and allow it to rest for 10 minutes.

When the chicken has been in the oven for about 15 minutes, start the ratatouille. Heat the olive oil in a large sauté pan over medium heat until shimmering. Add the garlic and cook for 30 seconds, then add the eggplant and ¼ teaspoon salt. Cook the eggplant until it is very soft and beginning to brown, 10 to 15 minutes. It will stick to the pan a little, thanks to the natural sugars caramelizing. If it begins to burn, loosen the eggplant by stirring gently and adding a teaspoon or two of water if necessary.

When the eggplant is very soft, add the zucchini, yellow squash, and bell pepper and cook until the vegetables are all very soft, about 10 minutes. The pan may still be sticky. If it looks like it's getting too dark, lower the heat.

Add the tomato paste and crushed tomatoes and cook for another 10 minutes, stirring and scraping the pan with a wooden spoon. All of the sticky bits on the bottom should release and be stirred into the ratatouille. Remove the pan from the heat and stir in the basil.

Carve the chicken into 8 pieces and serve over the ratatouille. Garnish with additional basil.

Nutritional analysis per serving: Calories: 550, Fat: 45 g, Saturated Fat: 8 g, Cholesterol: 125 mg, Fiber: 3 g, Protein: 27 g, Carbohydrates: 8 g, Sodium: 420 mg

Southwestern Chicken Wraps

Serves: 4

Prep Time:
15 minutes

Cook Time:
15 minutes

The star of this dish is the jalapeño pepper. Hot chiles are great detoxifiers as they contain potassium, magnesium, zinc, copper, vitamins A and C, and a phytonutrient called capsaicin, which gives your metabolism—and your taste buds!—a little kick.

- 4 (6-ounce) boneless, skinless chicken breasts
- ¾ teaspoon sea salt
- ¼ cup Mayonnaise (page 299) or Vegenaise
- ½ red onion, finely chopped
- 3 tablespoons chopped fresh cilantro, plus additional cilantro sprigs for serving
- grated zest and juice of 3 limes
- 2 jalapeños, seeded and minced
- 2 teaspoons ground cumin
- 1 romaine lettuce heart, separated into leaves
- 1 avocado, pitted, peeled, and thinly sliced
- lime wedges, for serving
- hot sauce, for serving (optional)

Put the chicken in a large saucepan. Fill it almost to the top with cold water and add ½ teaspoon of the salt. Bring the water to a boil over medium-high heat. Reduce the heat to a simmer and cook until the chicken is no longer pink in the center, 10 to 12 minutes.

Transfer the chicken to a cutting board. When cool enough to handle, shred the meat with your hands.

In a large bowl, combine the shredded chicken, mayonnaise, onion, chopped cilantro, lime zest and juice, jalapeños, cumin, and remaining ¼ teaspoon salt. Mix well.

Serve the chicken salad alongside lettuce leaves, avocado slices, cilantro sprigs, lime wedges, and hot sauce, if desired. Have your guests wrap the chicken salad in the lettuce leaves and top with garnishes, as desired.

Nutritional analysis per serving: *Calories: 360, Fat: 15 g, Saturated Fat: 3 g, Cholesterol: 112 mg, Fiber: 8 g, Protein: 40 g, Carbohydrates: 18 g, Sodium: 378 mg*

TOMATILLO CHICKEN

Serves: 4

Prep Time:
20 minutes

Cook Time:
40 minutes

This recipe is fun and suitable for little helpers. Have the kids test the tomatillo sauce after blending to make sure it tastes just right. Then, have them wash their hands and help you shred the chicken. Inviting kids to help prepare meals is a great way to convert picky eaters into adventurous diners.

- 1 medium yellow onion, quartered
- 2 large bone-in, skinless chicken breasts (or 4 [6 ounce] boneless, skinless chicken breasts if bone-in unavailable)
- ¾ teaspoon sea salt
- 3 large tomatillos, husked and quartered
- ½ cup toasted pepitas, plus more for garnish
- 1 bunch cilantro, plus additional chopped leaves for garnish
- 2 serrano chiles, seeded and chopped
- 1 garlic clove, halved
- 5 ounces baby kale
- 1 tablespoon grapeseed oil

Reserve one-quarter of the onion. Place the remaining onion and the chicken in a large saucepan. Add 4 cups of water and ½ teaspoon of the salt and bring to a boil. Reduce the heat to low and poach until the chicken is just cooked through, about 15 minutes. Transfer the chicken to a plate, discard the onion, and reserve the cooking liquid.

Place the tomatillos, pepitas, cilantro, chiles, garlic, reserved onion, 1 cup of the kale leaves, 1 cup of the chicken cooking liquid, and the remaining ¼ teaspoon salt in a blender. Puree until very smooth, 1 to 2 minutes.

Heat the oil in a large saucepan over medium-low heat. Add the tomatillo mixture; be careful, as it will splatter. Cook, stirring continuously, until thickened to a paste, about 10 minutes. Stir in 1½ cups of the chicken cooking liquid. Simmer, stirring occasionally, for 10 more minutes.

Pull the chicken meat from the bones and tear it into large chunks. Add the chicken and remaining kale to the pan and gently stir until the chicken is hot and the kale just wilts, about 1 minute.

Divide among four serving plates, garnish with pepitas and cilantro, and serve.

Nutritional analysis per serving: *Calories: 370, Fat: 18 g, Saturated Fat: 3 g, Cholesterol: 85 mg, Fiber: 4 g, Protein: 36 g, Carbohydrates: 16 g, Sodium: 488 mg*

Tuscan Chicken Cacciatore

Serves: 4

Prep Time:
15 minutes

Cook Time:
1 hour

I love inviting people over for dinner, and there is nothing easier than a one-pot meal when you are cooking for company. The next time you have extra friends and family members joining you at the table, simply double this recipe.

- 1 tablespoon coconut oil
- 1¼ pounds bone-in, skinless chicken thighs
- sea salt and freshly ground black pepper
- 2 medium yellow onions, chopped
- 2 red or green bell peppers, seeded and chopped
- 2 zucchini, diced
- 10 ounces button or cremini mushrooms, trimmed and halved
- 1 cup packed fresh basil leaves, plus 2 tablespoons chopped fresh basil for garnish
- 1 (28-ounce) can whole tomatoes
- ½ teaspoon dried thyme
- ½ teaspoon dried oregano

In a large Dutch oven, heat the oil over medium-high heat until shimmering. Season the chicken thighs with ¼ teaspoon salt and a pinch of black pepper. Brown the chicken in the hot oil, cooking for 3 to 4 minutes on each side. Transfer the chicken to a plate.

Add the onions and bell peppers to the pot and cook, stirring occasionally, until softened, about 10 minutes. Stir in the zucchini and mushrooms, and continue cooking for just a few minutes.

Add the basil leaves, stirring until wilted. Add the tomatoes with their juices, thyme, oregano, and ¼ teaspoon each salt and black pepper. Stir to combine, using the back of a wooden spoon to cut the tomatoes in half. Return the chicken to the pot and reduce the heat so the liquid is at a simmer. Cover and cook until the chicken is fully cooked, about 30 minutes.

Transfer the chicken to a plate and tent with foil to keep warm. Bring the vegetables and sauce to a boil over high heat and cook until about half of the liquid has evaporated, 5 to 8 minutes.

Serve the chicken with the vegetables and sauce, garnished with the chopped basil.

Nutritional analysis per serving: *Calories: 320, Fat: 10 g, Saturated Fat: 4.5 g, Cholesterol: 135 mg, Fiber: 5 g, Protein: 33 g, Carbohydrates: 24 g, Sodium: 460 mg*

YELLOW CURRY WITH CHICKEN MEATBALLS

Serves: 4

Prep Time:
30 minutes,
plus chilling
time

Cook Time:
20 minutes

Adding turmeric to your dishes is a great way to boost your intake of a powerful anti-inflammatory. The luscious curry served over these meatballs is light and refreshing but also creamy and satisfying.

- 1 large yellow onion, finely chopped
- 1 (2-inch) piece ginger, peeled and finely chopped
- 1 tablespoon plus 1 teaspoon yellow curry powder
- ¾ teaspoon sea salt
- 1 pound ground chicken
- 4 lemongrass stalks, roughly chopped
- juice of 2 limes, plus grated zest of 1 lime
- 1 teaspoon ground turmeric
- 2 cups low-sodium chicken stock
- 1 cup full-fat unsweetened coconut milk
- 1 red bell pepper, seeded and finely chopped
- 1 jalapeño, seeded and finely chopped
- 1 bunch cilantro (including stems), finely chopped

In a large bowl, combine 2 tablespoons of the onion, 1 tablespoon of the ginger, 1 tablespoon of the curry powder, and ½ teaspoon of the salt. Add the chicken and mix gently with your hands until well combined. Cover the bowl and refrigerate for 15 to 20 minutes.

In a food processor, pulse the lemongrass until very finely minced, with no bristly strands remaining, scraping the bowl occasionally. Transfer to a large saucepan. Add the remaining ginger and onion, the lime juice and zest, the turmeric, and the remaining 1 teaspoon curry powder. Stir in the chicken stock and coconut milk and bring to a boil over medium-high heat. Reduce the heat to medium to maintain a steady simmer.

Form the chilled chicken mixture into 1-inch balls. Carefully drop them into the simmering curry. Adjust the heat to maintain a simmer and simmer until the meatballs are cooked through, about 15 minutes. Season with the remaining ¼ teaspoon salt.

Fold most of the bell pepper, jalapeño, and cilantro into the curry sauce, reserving a small amount of each for garnish. Simmer until just heated through, about 2 minutes. Divide among four serving bowls, garnish with the reserved bell pepper, jalapeño, and cilantro, and serve.

Nutritional analysis per serving: *Calories: 332, Fat: 22 g, Saturated Fat: 13 g, Cholesterol: 98 mg, Fiber: 2 g, Protein: 23 g, Carbohydrates: 13 g, Sodium: 459 mg*

Red Curry Stew with Chicken and Eggplant

Serves: 4

Prep Time:
20 minutes

Cook Time:
45 minutes

Here is another one-pot meal you will be thankful to have in your meal plan rotation. This hearty stew has just the right amount of heat, but feel free to add a pinch of cayenne if you want even more spice.

- 1 tablespoon coconut oil
- 1 pound boneless, skinless chicken thighs
- sea salt and freshly ground black pepper
- ½ medium red onion, sliced
- 1 teaspoon chili powder
- 1 teaspoon grated fresh ginger
- 1 (13.5-ounce) can full-fat unsweetened coconut milk
- 1 large eggplant, diced
- 1 zucchini, diced
- 3 or 4 red Thai chiles, seeded and halved lengthwise
- 2 pints cherry or grape tomatoes
- 8 ounces green beans, trimmed and cut into 2-inch pieces
- 2 scallions, chopped
- ⅓ cup chopped fresh cilantro
- grated zest of 1 lime
- juice of 2 limes
- 3 tablespoons chopped almonds

In a large sauté pan, heat ½ tablespoon of the coconut oil over medium-high heat until shimmering. Season the chicken thighs with ¼ teaspoon salt and a pinch of black pepper and add them to the pan. Brown the chicken in the hot oil, cooking for 2 to 3 minutes per side. Transfer the chicken to a plate.

Add the remaining ½ tablespoon coconut oil to the sauté pan. Add the onion and sauté until softened, about 5 minutes.

Add the chili powder and ginger and cook, stirring constantly, for just 30 seconds. Add the coconut milk and ¾ cup of water and stir to combine. Stir in the eggplant, zucchini, Thai chiles, and ¼ teaspoon each salt and black pepper. Return the chicken to the pan. Bring the liquid to a boil, cover, and reduce the heat so the stew stays at a simmer. Cook until the chicken is cooked through, about 20 minutes.

Add the tomatoes and green beans and stir to combine. Continue to simmer, uncovered, for 10 minutes.

Remove the pan from the heat. Stir in the scallions, cilantro, and lime zest and juice. Remove the Thai chiles from the dish (if desired), garnish with the almonds, and serve.

Nutritional analysis per serving: *Calories: 510, Fat: 33 g, Saturated Fat: 23 g, Cholesterol: 135 mg, Fiber: 9 g, Protein: 30 g, Carbohydrates: 26 g, Sodium: 450 mg*

Ginger-Lemon Chicken with Spinach

Serves: 4

Prep Time:
20 minutes

Cook Time:
1 hour

This is a true chicken dish for the soul. When you are feeling a bit run down and need a nourishing meal to warm you from the inside out, look no further than your kitchen and this recipe to nurture your body, mind, and spirit.

- 1 (2-inch) piece ginger, peeled and minced
- sea salt
- 3 tablespoons grapeseed oil
- 1 (3½-pound) whole chicken
- 2 lemons, 1 sliced into thin rounds, 1 cut into wedges for serving
- 9 ounces baby spinach
- ¼ teaspoon crushed red pepper flakes

Preheat the oven to 425°F.

In a small bowl, use a spoon to mash together the ginger, 2 table-spoons salt, and 2 tablespoons of the oil. Set aside.

Pat the chicken dry with paper towels. Using your fingers, gently loosen the skin from the chicken breasts. Being careful not to tear the skin, spread half of the ginger-salt paste evenly between the skin and meat; pat the skin back down. Rub the remaining paste inside the chicken cavity. Tuck the entire sliced lemon into the cavity (you may have to cut a few slices in half).

Tie the chicken legs together with cotton kitchen twine; tuck the wing tips underneath. Rub the chicken with the remaining 1 tablespoon oil. Place the chicken, breast-side up, in a roasting pan.

Roast the chicken, occasionally basting with the pan juices, until golden-brown, 50 to 55 minutes; an instant-read thermometer inserted in the thickest part of the thigh should read 165°F. Transfer the chicken to a cutting board and tent with foil, reserving the hot baking sheet; allow the chicken to rest for 10 minutes before carving.

Scatter the spinach over the pan juices on the baking sheet. Place the pan back in the oven until the spinach has begun to wilt, 2 to 3 minutes.

Toss the spinach on the hot pan until it is fully wilted and dressed with pan juices. Season with a pinch of salt and the red pepper flakes. Carve the chicken and serve with the spinach and lemon wedges on the side.

Nutritional analysis per serving: *Calories: 480, Fat: 36 g, Saturated Fat: 8 g, Cholesterol: 128 mg, Fiber: 2 g, Protein: 34 g, Carbohydrates: 5 g, Sodium: 460 mg*

MOROCCAN-STYLE CHICKEN

Serves: 6

Prep Time:
20 minutes

Cook Time:
40 minutes

The blend of spices in this dish creates aromatic, authentic Moroccan flavors with no tagine necessary! The lemon loses its acidic tartness in the oven, adding savory depth to the sauce with just a bright zing at the finish. Pair with Green Beans and Almonds (page 254).

- 1 tablespoon fennel seeds
- 1 tablespoon cumin seeds
- 2 teaspoons coriander seeds
- 1 teaspoon ground cinnamon
- 1 teaspoon paprika
- ½ teaspoon Aleppo pepper or ¼ teaspoon crushed red pepper flakes
- 1 teaspoon sea salt
- 2 tablespoons plus 1 teaspoon extra-virgin olive oil
- 3 small fennel bulbs, each cut into 8 wedges, fronds reserved
- 3 medium shallots, sliced
- 6 (4-ounce) boneless, skinless chicken thighs
- 1 lemon, very thinly sliced and seeded
- ¼ cup finely chopped green olives
- 2 large tomatoes, diced

Preheat the oven to 475°F.

In a small skillet, heat the fennel, cumin, and coriander seeds over medium heat, tossing occasionally, until fragrant and toasted, about 3 minutes. Cool, then transfer to a spice grinder and coarsely grind. Transfer the spices to a large bowl and stir in the cinnamon, paprika, pepper, ¾ teaspoon of the salt, and 2 tablespoons of the oil. Add the fennel wedges, shallots, and chicken and mix until everything is evenly coated.

Spread the chicken and vegetables evenly on a large rimmed baking sheet. Roast until the chicken is cooked through and the vegetables are tender, about 40 minutes.

Meanwhile, toss the lemon slices with the remaining 1 teaspoon oil until well coated. Spread in a single layer on a second baking sheet. Roast alongside the chicken until golden brown and tender, about 30 minutes. Transfer the lemons to a cutting board. When cool enough to handle, chop very finely (including the peel) and transfer to a medium bowl.

Finely chop the reserved fennel fronds. Add half of the chopped fronds to the lemons and mix in the olives, tomatoes, and remaining ¼ teaspoon salt.

Divide the chicken and roasted vegetables among six serving plates and drizzle with the pan juices. Spoon the tomato mixture on top, garnish with the remaining chopped fennel fronds, and serve.

Nutritional analysis per serving: Calories: 250, Fat: 11 g, Saturated Fat: 2 g, Cholesterol: 110 mg, Fiber: 6 g, Protein: 25 g, Carbohydrates: 15 g, Sodium: 522 mg

COCONUT CURRY CHICKEN SOUP WITH ALMONDS

Serves: 4

Prep Time:
15 minutes

Cook Time:
30 minutes

Each ingredient in this soup contains immune-boosting nutrients and phytonu-trients that prevent disease. Double the batch and freeze half so that you have soup on hand the next time someone you love is feeling under the weather.

- 1 tablespoon coconut oil
- 3 medium shallots, thinly sliced
- 2 to 3 teaspoons mild curry powder
- ½ teaspoon ground turmeric
- ½ teaspoon ground ginger
- ¼ teaspoon sea salt
- ¼ teaspoon freshly ground black pepper
- 4 cups low-sodium chicken stock
- 1 pound thin-cut chicken cutlets
- 1 (13.5-ounce) can full-fat unsweetened coconut milk
- 1 cup sliced shiitake mushroom caps
- 1 cup sliced sugar snap peas
- 1 red bell pepper, seeded and chopped
- ½ cup chopped fresh cilantro
- 2 scallions, chopped
- juice of 2 limes
- ¼ cup sliced almonds
- 1 teaspoon toasted sesame oil

In a medium stockpot, heat the oil over medium-high heat until shim-mering. Add the shallots and sauté until translucent, 3 to 4 minutes.

Stir in 2 teaspoons of the curry powder, the turmeric, ginger, salt, and black pepper and cook for 30 seconds. Pour in the chicken stock and 1 cup of water; stir to combine. Bring the liquid to a boil over high heat.

Add the chicken cutlets, trying to make sure they are submerged in the liquid. Reduce to a simmer and cook until the chicken is cooked through, 10 to 15 minutes (cut into one of the thicker cutlets to verify that it is no longer pink inside). Transfer the chicken cutlets to a bowl and let cool.

Add the coconut milk, mushrooms, sugar snap peas, and red bell pepper to the pot. Let the soup continue to simmer for 7 to 10 minutes. Taste and add more curry powder, if desired.

Meanwhile, cut the chicken into bite-size pieces. Remove the soup from the heat and stir in the chicken, cilantro, scallions, and lime juice. Ladle the soup into four bowls. Garnish with almonds, drizzle with sesame oil, and serve.

Nutritional analysis per serving: *Calories: 480, Fat: 33 g, Saturated Fat: 23 g, Cholesterol: 100 mg, Fiber: 3 g, Protein: 35 g, Carbohydrates: 15 g, Sodium: 351 mg*

SOUTHWESTERN TURKEY CHILI

Serves: 8

Prep Time:
20 minutes

Cook Time:
30 minutes

This chili will flood your body with a healthy dose of potassium, an important blood pressure regulator. Most SAD (standard American diet) consumers don't get enough potassium due to the lack of fruits and vegetables in their diet. Not only will this dish help your body relax and work more effectively, but the aromas and flavors will put you in that cozy place that home-cooked meals provide.

- 1 tablespoon extra-virgin olive oil
- 2 pounds ground turkey, preferably dark meat
- 1 yellow onion, finely chopped
- 2 bell peppers (any color), seeded and finely chopped
- 2 jalapeños, seeded and minced
- 6 garlic cloves, minced
- 3 tablespoons chili powder
- 1½ tablespoons smoked paprika
- 1½ tablespoons ground cumin
- 1½ tablespoons garlic powder
- sea salt and freshly ground black pepper
- 1 (28-ounce) can tomato puree
- 1 (28-ounce) can diced tomatoes
- 1 avocado, pitted, peeled, and sliced, for garnish
- 2 tablespoons chopped fresh cilantro, for garnish
- 1 scallion, sliced, for garnish

In a large saucepan, heat the oil over medium-high heat until shimmering. Add the turkey and cook, breaking up with a spoon, until no longer pink, 5 to 7 minutes.

Stir in the onion, bell peppers, jalapeños, garlic, chili powder, paprika, cumin, garlic powder, 1 teaspoon salt, and a pinch of black pepper. Add the tomato puree and the diced tomatoes with their juices, reduce the heat to medium, and cook, stirring occasionally, for 20 to 25 minutes.

Serve, topped with avocado, cilantro, and scallions.

Nutritional analysis per serving: *Calories: 310, Fat: 16 g, Saturated Fat: 3.5 g, Cholesterol: 85 mg, Fiber: 6 g, Protein: 25 g, Carbohydrates: 21 g, Sodium: 460 mg*

SPICED TURKEY AND ZUCCHINI MEATBALLS

Ground turkey makes for tasty meatballs, meatloaf, burgers, or chili. Choose dark meat for this recipe, as it will retain more moisture and yield a juicier meatball. Pair with a vegetable side dish such as Mashed Cauliflower with Horseradish (page 265).

- 1 pound ground turkey (preferably dark meat)
- 1 small zucchini, grated
- 2 tablespoons minced shallot
- 1 garlic clove, minced
- 1 large omega-3 egg, beaten
- 1 teaspoon dried oregano
- ¾ teaspoon sea salt
- ½ teaspoon Aleppo pepper or ¼ teaspoon crushed red pepper flakes
- ½ teaspoon fennel seeds, minced or crushed
- ½ teaspoon dried sage
- 2 tablespoons grapeseed oil, plus more if needed
- chopped fresh basil or chives, for garnish

Preheat the oven to 400°F.

In a large bowl, combine all of the ingredients except the grapeseed oil and basil and mix well. Using wet hands, form the mixture into 12 balls, each about the size of a tangerine.

Heat the grapeseed oil in a large oven-safe sauté pan over medium-high heat until shimmering. Place the meatballs in the hot pan, leaving space between them. (Depending on the size of your sauté pan, you may need to cook the meatballs in batches.) Cook, using a large spoon to turn the meatballs gently, until brown, about 30 seconds per side. The meatballs will be soft, so turn carefully.

Transfer the sauté pan to the oven and bake until the meatballs feel firm to the touch, 8 to 10 minutes. Garnish with basil and serve.

Nutritional analysis per serving: *Calories: 262, Fat: 19 g, Saturated Fat: 5 g, Cholesterol: 145 mg, Fiber: 1 g, Protein: 21 g, Carbohydrates: 2 g, Sodium: 520 mg*

CHILI-SPICED TURKEY MEATLOAF WITH ROASTED CARROT SALAD

Serves: 8

Prep Time: 20 minutes

Cook Time: 1 hour

Protein keeps the nighttime munchies at bay. If you tend to feel hungry or have a habit of grazing after dinner, this meal will help you meet your intake of nutritious protein, which keeps your blood sugar stable and prevents cravings.

- 6 garlic cloves, halved
- 2 celery ribs, coarsely chopped
- 1 small yellow onion, coarsely chopped
- ½ cup coconut flour
- 3 large omega-3 eggs, beaten
- 3 tablespoons paprika
- 1 tablespoon chili powder
- sea salt
- 2 pounds ground turkey (preferably dark meat)
- 2 pounds carrots, peeled and cut into steak fries
- 2 tablespoons plus 2 teaspoons grapeseed oil
- ½ cup pepitas
- ½ cup chopped fresh cilantro
- ½ teaspoon ground cumin

Preheat the oven to 375°F.

In the bowl of a food processor, pulse the garlic, celery, and onion until very finely chopped. Transfer the vegetables to a large bowl and add the coconut flour, eggs, 1 tablespoon of the paprika, the chili powder, and 1 teaspoon salt. Add the turkey and, using your hands, mix until combined; do not overmix or the meatloaf will be dense.

Gently pat the meat into a loaf and place in an 8½-by-4½-inch loaf pan. Do not press down or into the corners. Place the pan on a rimmed baking sheet and bake on the top rack for 50 minutes.

While the meatloaf cooks, toss the carrots with 2 teaspoons of the oil and a pinch of salt on two large rimmed baking sheets. Roast on the bottom and middle racks of the oven, tossing once halfway through, until tender, 15 to 20 minutes. Remove and tent with foil to keep warm.

When the meatloaf has baked for 50 minutes, stir together the remaining 2 tablespoons paprika and 2 tablespoons grapeseed oil. Brush the top of the loaf with the mixture and continue cooking until an instant-read thermometer inserted into the thickest part of the loaf registers 155°F, about 10 more minutes. Remove from the oven; let rest for 10 minutes before slicing.

While the meatloaf rests, place the pepitas in a small skillet and lightly toast them over medium-low heat, stirring frequently, until they take on the slightest hint of color, 3 to 5 minutes.

Combine the carrots, pepitas, cilantro, and cumin, tossing to combine. Serve with the meatloaf.

Nutritional analysis per serving: *Calories: 395, Fat: 23 g, Saturated Fat: 5 g, Cholesterol: 168 mg, Fiber: 8 g, Protein: 29 g, Carbohydrates: 20 g, Sodium: 521 mg*

ROASTED TURKEY WITH HERB PASTE

Serves: 6

Prep Time:
20 minutes

Cook Time:
1 hour

If you are like me and wish Thanksgiving came around monthly instead of yearly, then you will love this recipe. Just when I thought nothing could top my favorite Thanksgiving turkey, I found this recipe and now enjoy making it all year round because it is simple yet elegant. Serve with a side of Cauliflower "Rice" (page 264).

- 1 (1-pound) boneless, skinless turkey breast
- ¼ teaspoon sea salt
- ¼ teaspoon freshly ground black pepper
- 2 scallions, roughly chopped
- 2 garlic cloves, halved
- 1 cup fresh parsley leaves
- leaves from 4 to 6 thyme sprigs
- leaves from 1 large rosemary sprig
- 1 tablespoon Dijon mustard
- 1 tablespoon extra-virgin olive oil
- 1 lemon, sliced into 6 rounds

Preheat the oven to 350°F.

Place the turkey breast in a baking dish and season with the salt and black pepper.

In the bowl of a food processor, combine the scallions, garlic, parsley, thyme, rosemary, mustard, and olive oil. Pulse until a thick paste forms, 30 seconds to 1 minute.

Spread one-half to two-thirds of the herb paste over the top of the turkey breast. Layer the lemon slices over the herb paste.

Roast the turkey until an instant-read thermometer inserted into the thickest part reads 165°F, 45 to 60 minutes. Remove the turkey from the oven, tent with foil, and let rest for 10 to 15 minutes.

Remove the lemon slices and slice the turkey. Arrange the turkey slices on a platter and top with additional herb paste. Serve.

Nutritional analysis per serving: *Calories: 231, Fat: 7 g, Saturated Fat: 1 g, Cholesterol: 60 mg, Fiber: 2 g, Protein: 36 g, Carbohydrates: 3 g, Sodium: 230 mg*

TURKEY BURGERS

Serves: 4

Prep Time:
20 minutes

Cook Time:
15 minutes

For a heartier meal, try pairing these burgers with Onion-Leek Soup (page 126).

- ¼ cup apple cider vinegar
- ¾ teaspoon sea salt
- ½ teaspoon freshly ground black pepper
- 12 ounces radishes, very thinly sliced
- 1 teaspoon fresh lime juice
- 2 tablespoons Mayonnaise (page 299) or Vegenaise
- 1 pound ground turkey
- 1 large zucchini, coarsely grated
- 1 bunch chives, thinly sliced
- 1 large omega-3 egg, beaten
- 1 teaspoon ancho chile powder
- 1 teaspoon ground cumin
- ¼ teaspoon cayenne pepper
- 2 tablespoons grapeseed oil
- 16 red lettuce leaves
- 2 tomatoes, thinly sliced

Combine the vinegar and ¼ teaspoon each of the salt and black pepper in a medium bowl. Add the radishes, turn to coat, and let stand.

In a small bowl, whisk the lime juice into the mayonnaise; set aside.

Combine the turkey, zucchini, chives (reserve a little for the garnish), egg, chile, cumin, cayenne, and remaining ½ teaspoon salt and ¼ teaspoon black pepper in a large bowl. Form into 4 equal-size patties.

Heat the oil in a large nonstick skillet over medium heat until shimmering. Add the patties and cook, turning once, until cooked through, about 15 minutes.

For each serving, stack 2 lettuce leaves and place 1 burger in the center. Top each burger with some of the lime-mayo mixture, tomato slices, pickled radishes, and reserved chives. Sandwich with 2 more lettuce leaves and serve with any remaining radishes on the side.

Nutritional analysis per serving: *Calories: 340, Fat: 20 g, Saturated Fat: 4 g, Cholesterol: 130 mg, Fiber: 4 g, Protein: 27 g, Carbohydrates: 14 g, Sodium: 481 mg*

TURKEY PICCATA WITH BRUSSELS SPROUT LEAVES AND BROCCOLI RABE

The capers are what make a piccata memorable—they're salty and pungent and stimulate your palate so that you enjoy all the fresh flavors of this dish. The traditional piccata is made from veal cutlets breaded in flour, which takes away from the otherwise healthy nature of the dish. You can enjoy this updated version without sabotaging your health.

- 2 bunches broccoli rabe, trimmed and cut into 2-inch pieces
- 1 pound Brussels sprouts
- 4 tablespoons extra-virgin olive oil
- 3 garlic cloves, minced
- sea salt and freshly ground black pepper
- 1¼ pounds thin-cut turkey cutlets
- 2 tablespoons fresh lemon juice
- 1 tablespoon rinsed, finely chopped capers
- 2 tablespoons chopped fresh parsley

Bring a large pot of water to a boil over high heat. Cook the broccoli rabe until tender, about 3 minutes. Drain in a colander.

Remove the leaves of the Brussels sprouts by trimming the end of each one and halving it. Remove as many leaves as you can, saving the cores for vegetable stock. Reserve the leaves.

In a large nonstick sauté pan, warm 1 tablespoon of the oil over medium-high heat until shimmering. Cook the Brussels sprout leaves, stirring constantly, for about 6 minutes. Stir in the broccoli rabe and cook until the Brussels sprout leaves are tender, 2 to 3 minutes. Stir in the garlic, ¼ teaspoon salt, and a pinch of black pepper and cook for about 1 minute. Transfer the vegetables from the pan to a bowl; tent with foil to keep warm.

Wipe out the pan. Warm ½ tablespoon of the oil over medium-high heat until shimmering. Season the turkey with ¼ teaspoon each salt and black pepper. Sauté the turkey until browned and fully cooked, 2 to 3 minutes per side. Transfer the turkey to a platter.

Heat the remaining 2½ tablespoons oil over medium heat. Add the lemon juice, capers, and 1 tablespoon of water, stirring and using a spatula to scrape up any browned turkey bits in the pan. Spoon the mixture over the turkey breasts. Garnish with parsley and serve with the reserved vegetables on the side.

Nutritional analysis per serving: Calories: 360, Fat: 16 g, Saturated Fat: 2.5 g, Cholesterol: 80 mg, Fiber: 6 g, Protein: 39 g, Carbohydrates: 17 g, Sodium: 470 mg

Thai Chicken Noodle Soup (page 130)

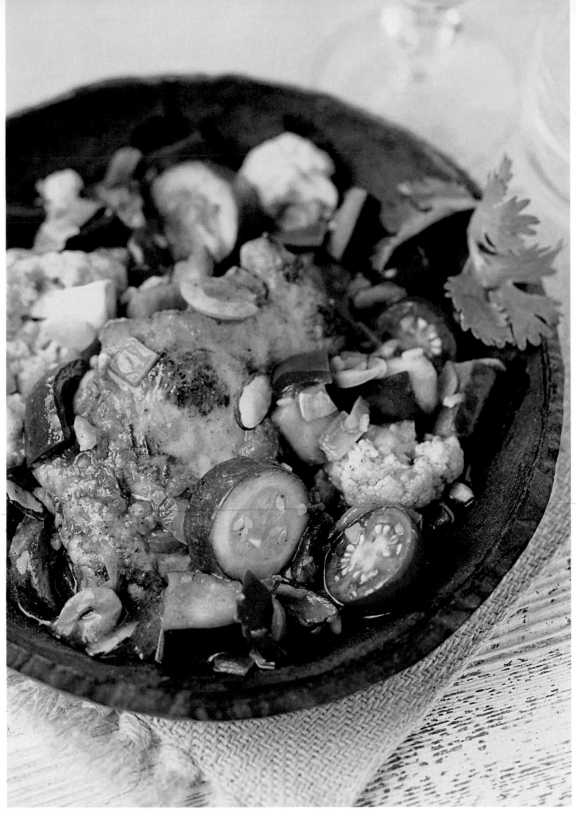

Moroccan Chicken and Vegetable Stew (page 175)

Chicken with Oven-Roasted Tomatoes (page 183)

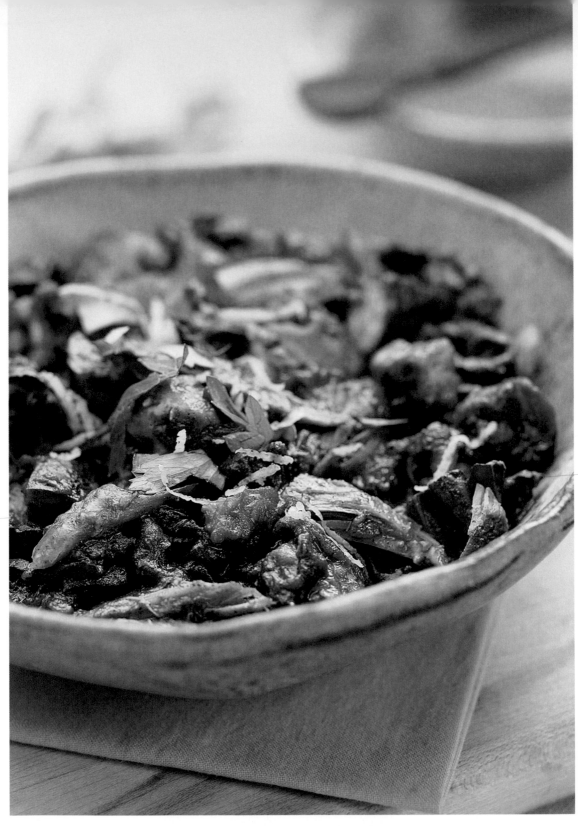

Lebanese-Style Lamb Stew (page 247)

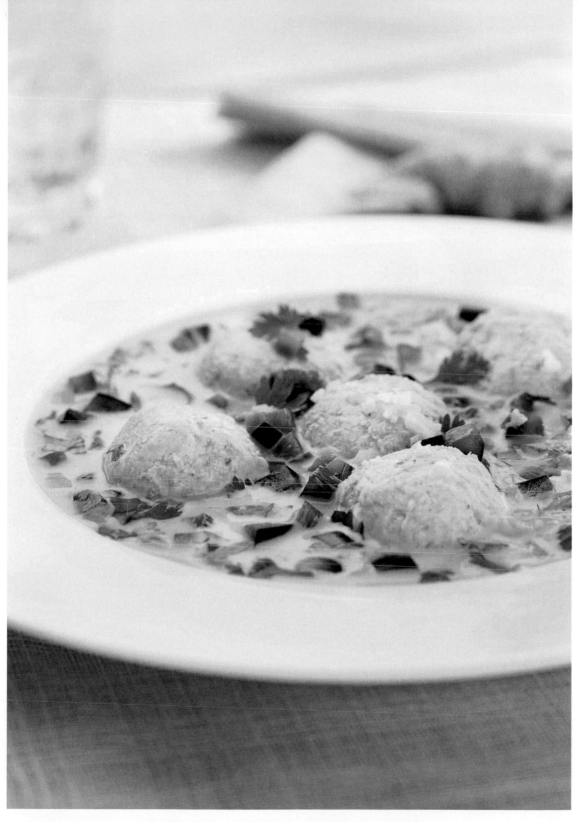

Yellow Curry with Chicken Meatballs (page 198)

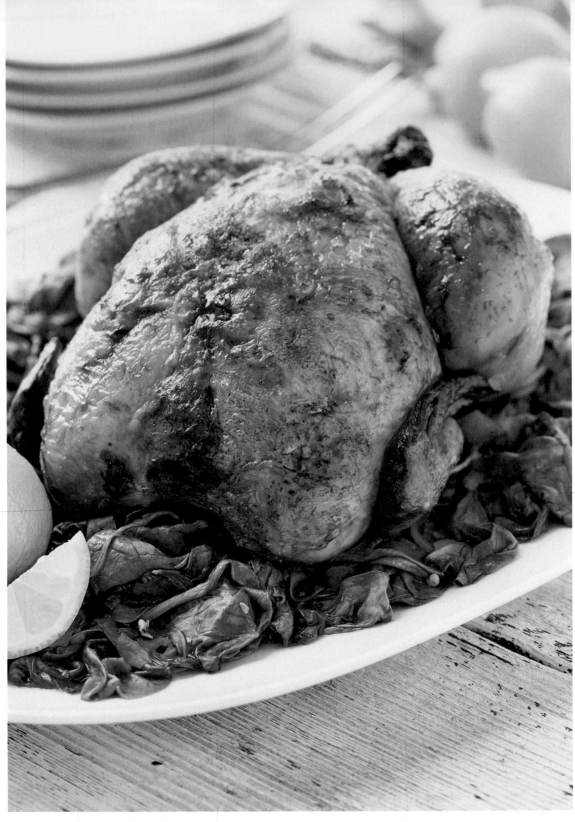

Ginger–Lemon Chicken with Spinach (page 202)

Turkey Burgers (page 213)

Slow-Cooked Short Ribs with Celery Root Puree (page 231)

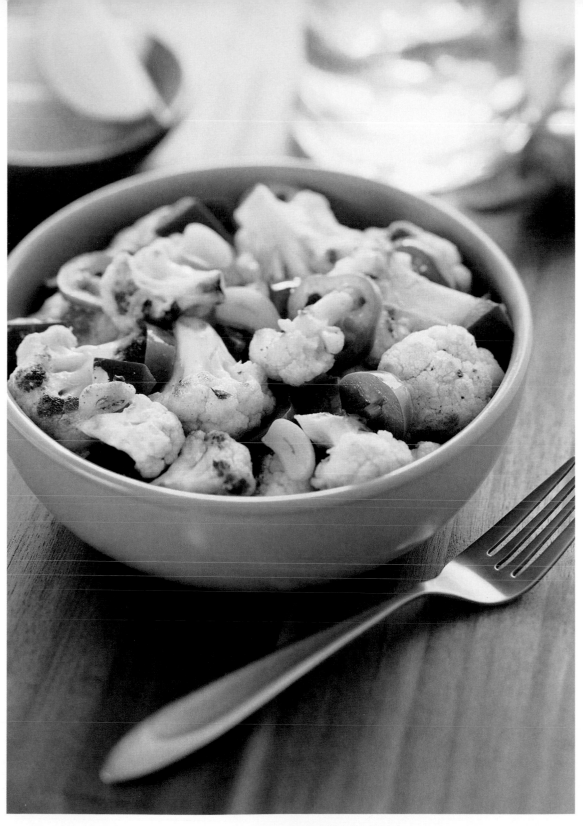

Spicy Cauliflower Sauté (page 259)

Broccoli Rabe with Hot Italian Sausage (page 263)

Jicama Fries (page 271)

Deviled Eggs (page 274)

Egg Salad in Endive Spears (page 275)

Stuffed Campari Tomatoes (page 276)

Creamy Herbed Tahini Dip (page 281)

Gremolata with Almonds (page 292)

Meat

BEEF CHILI

Higher in omega-3 fatty acids than feedlot beef, as well as in other compounds known to reduce weight such as CLA (conjugated linoleic acids), grass-fed beef is tasty and becoming more widely available as consumers increase demand for better quality meat.

Serves: 4

Prep Time: 30 minutes

Cook Time: 3 to 3½ hours

- 1 tablespoon extra-virgin olive oil
- 1 pound grass-fed beef stew meat, cut into 1-inch pieces
- 2 medium yellow onions, chopped
- 2 green or red bell peppers, seeded and chopped
- 4 celery ribs, chopped
- 2 zucchini, diced
- 2 garlic cloves, minced
- 1 tablespoon tomato paste
- 2 canned chipotle peppers in adobo sauce, seeded and chopped, plus 2 teaspoons adobo sauce
- 1 teaspoon ground cumin
- 1 teaspoon chili powder
- ½ teaspoon ground cinnamon
- ¼ teaspoon sea salt
- ¼ teaspoon freshly ground black pepper
- 1 (28-ounce) can whole tomatoes
- ¼ cup low-sodium chicken stock
- ½ cup chopped fresh cilantro, for garnish
- ¼ cup sliced radishes, for garnish
- ½ avocado, pitted, peeled, and chopped, for garnish

In a Dutch oven, warm ½ tablespoon of the oil over medium-high heat until shimmering. Add the beef and cook until browned, about 3 minutes per side. Using a slotted spoon, transfer the beef to a bowl.

Add the remaining ½ tablespoon oil to the pot. Sauté the onions and bell peppers for 6 minutes. Add the celery and zucchini and sauté for another 5 minutes. If the vegetables are browning too much, reduce the heat to medium.

Stir in the garlic, tomato paste, chipotle peppers, adobo sauce, cumin, chili powder, cinnamon, salt, and black pepper. Cook for 30 seconds before adding the tomatoes with their juices and the chicken stock. Use the back of a wooden spoon to break the tomatoes in half. Bring to a boil, then reduce the heat to low so the mixture is at a simmer.

Return the meat to the pot, cover, and cook, stirring occasionally, until the meat is tender, 2½ to 3 hours. Taste and adjust the seasonings to make it spicier, if desired. Ladle the chili into bowls. Garnish with cilantro, radishes, and avocado and serve.

Nutritional analysis per serving: *Calories: 320, Fat: 11 g, Saturated Fat: 2.5 g, Cholesterol: 60 mg, Fiber: 8 g, Protein: 31 g, Carbohydrates: 26 g, Sodium: 310 mg*

SLOW-COOKED BRISKET WITH FENNEL AND ONIONS

Serves: 4

Prep Time:
30 minutes

Cook Time: 8
to 10 hours
(unattended)
plus 10 minutes

Make this a zero-fuss meal by prepping it Sunday night. Before leaving for the day on Monday morning, simply turn on your slow cooker and let the aroma of herbs, spices, and savory meat permeate your home. Walk in, enjoy the comforts of a truly slow-cooked meal, and marvel at the simplicity of living well. (If you don't have a slow cooker, you can cook the stew for about 1 hour in a covered Dutch oven set over medium heat.)

- 2 tablespoons cider vinegar
- 2 fennel bulbs, halved and sliced
- 2 yellow onions, halved and sliced
- 1 (16-ounce) can diced tomatoes
- 1 head garlic, cloves peeled
- 8 to 10 thyme sprigs
- 1 (3-pound) grass-fed lean brisket, cut into 4 pieces
- 2 teaspoons chili powder
- ½ teaspoon sea salt
- ¼ teaspoon freshly ground black pepper
- chopped fresh parsley, for garnish

Pour the vinegar and ½ cup of water into a 6-quart slow cooker.

In a large bowl, combine the fennel, onions, diced tomatoes with their juices, garlic, and thyme. Transfer half of the vegetable mixture to the slow cooker.

Season the brisket all over with the chili powder, salt, and black pepper. Place the pieces of meat on top of the vegetables in the slow cooker. Pour the remaining vegetables on top.

Cook on low until the meat easily pulls apart with a fork, 8 to 10 hours. Let the brisket rest, covered, for about 30 minutes. Remove the thyme sprigs.

Using a ladle, transfer 3 cups of the cooking liquid to a medium sauté pan. Bring to a boil over high heat and let the liquid reduce until it thickens into a gravy—keeping a careful eye on it so it doesn't over-reduce or burn—8 to 10 minutes. Remove from the heat.

Slice the brisket against the grain. Pour the gravy over the brisket slices, garnish with the parsley, and serve with the vegetables on the side.

Nutritional analysis per serving: Calories: 300, Fat: 11 g, Saturated Fat: 4 g, Cholesterol: 76 mg, Fiber: 7 g, Protein: 27 g, Carbohydrates: 25 g, Sodium: 486 mg

ASIAN-STYLE BEEF STEW

Surprise your family with this Asian-style take on the traditional beef stew. It's comfort food at its tastiest — and healthiest.

- 1¼ pounds grass-fed beef stew meat, cut into 1-inch pieces
- 1 large daikon radish, peeled and cut into 1-inch pieces
- 4 scallions, white parts cut into 2-inch lengths, green parts thinly sliced
- 2 tablespoons minced fresh ginger
- 3 tablespoons brown (*hatcho*) miso
- 2 small zucchini, diced
- 2 small yellow summer squash, diced
- 7 ounces enoki mushrooms, trimmed and separated into smaller pieces
- ½ teaspoon freshly ground black pepper

Serves: 4

Prep Time: 15 minutes

Cook Time: 1 hour and 45 minutes

Combine the beef, daikon, scallion whites, and ginger in a large saucepan. Add 4 cups of water; the water should just cover the ingredients. Bring to a boil over high heat. Skim and discard any foam that accumulates on the surface.

Meanwhile, whisk the miso with ½ cup of warm water in a small bowl. Stir into the pot, reduce the heat to low, cover, and simmer until the beef is very tender, about 1½ hours.

Gently fold in the zucchini, squash, mushrooms, and black pepper. Simmer until the squash are crisp-tender, about 10 minutes. Ladle into four soup bowls, garnish with the scallion greens, and serve.

Nutritional analysis per serving: *Calories: 513, Fat: 28 g, Saturated Fat: 11 g, Cholesterol: 164 mg, Fiber: 5 g, Protein: 46 g, Carbohydrates: 19 g, Sodium: 551 mg*

BAKED MEATBALLS WITH CAULIFLOWER PUREE

Serves: 4

Prep Time:
30 minutes

Cook Time:
50 minutes

This is a sumptuous meal without the expense of a fancy restaurant! Feel free to substitute ground turkey for the grass-fed beef in this recipe for a little variety.

- 1 pound ground grass-fed beef
- 4 button mushrooms, minced
- 1 large omega-3 egg, beaten
- 3 teaspoons minced garlic
- 2 tablespoons minced shallot
- 2 tablespoons coarsely chopped pine nuts
- ½ teaspoon dried thyme
- ½ teaspoon dried oregano
- ½ teaspoon crushed red pepper flakes
- sea salt and freshly ground black pepper
- 2 tablespoons grapeseed oil
- 1 small head cauliflower, coarsely chopped
- ¼ cup unsweetened almond milk
- ¼ cup plus 1 tablespoon extra-virgin olive oil
- 1 small yellow onion, minced
- 1 teaspoon tomato paste
- 2 cups canned tomato puree
- 1 bunch kale, stemmed and finely shredded

Preheat the oven to 400°F.

In a large mixing bowl, combine the beef, mushrooms, egg, 2 teaspoons of the garlic, the shallot, pine nuts, thyme, oregano, red pepper flakes, ¼ teaspoon salt, and a pinch of black pepper. Mix well. Using wet hands, form the mixture into 12 balls, each about the size of a tangerine.

Heat the grapeseed oil in a large oven-safe sauté pan over medium-high heat until shimmering. Place the meatballs in the hot pan, leaving space between them. (Depending on the size of your sauté pan, you may need to cook the meatballs in batches.) Cook, using a large spoon to turn the meatballs gently, until brown, about 30 seconds per side. The meatballs will be soft, so turn carefully.

Transfer the sauté pan to the oven and bake until the meatballs feel firm to the touch, 8 to 10 minutes. Transfer them to a plate.

While the meatballs bake, pour 1 cup of water into the bottom of a medium saucepan and bring it to a boil over high heat. Place a steaming rack or basket over the boiling water. Add the cauliflower, cover, and steam until it is very soft and easily breaks apart, about 10 minutes.

Transfer the cauliflower to a food processor or blender and add the almond milk, ¼ cup of the olive oil, and ¼ teaspoon salt. Puree until very smooth, then transfer the puree to a large oven-safe baking dish or gratin dish. Set aside.

In a large saucepan, heat the remaining 1 tablespoon olive oil over medium-low heat. Add the onion and remaining 1 teaspoon garlic and sauté until they begin to brown, about 5 minutes. Add the tomato paste and cook for 1 minute. Add the tomato puree and ¼ teaspoon salt and bring to a simmer; reduce the heat to low and cook for 15 minutes. Stir in the shredded kale and cook until the kale is very tender, about 5 minutes.

Arrange the meatballs on top of the cauliflower puree, then ladle the tomato sauce over the meatballs. Place the baking dish in the oven and bake for 10 minutes.

Serve each guest 3 meatballs, along with some cauliflower puree and tomato-kale sauce.

Nutritional analysis per serving: *Calories: 499, Fat: 36 g, Saturated Fat: 6 g, Cholesterol: 140 mg, Fiber: 6 g, Protein: 29 g, Carbohydrates: 23 g, Sodium: 580 mg*

Serves: 4

Prep Time:
20 minutes

Cook Time:
30 minutes

Chipotle-Rubbed Steak Salad
with Onions and Peppers

Chipotle chiles are dried, smoked red jalapeños. If you can't find chipotle in powdered form, you can use ancho chile powder or smoked paprika.

- 1½ pounds grass-fed beef steaks (such as rib-eye, strip, or hanger)
- 1 tablespoon chipotle chile powder
- 1 teaspoon sea salt
- ¼ teaspoon ground cumin
- ¼ teaspoon ground coriander
- 2 tablespoons extra-virgin olive oil
- 2 garlic cloves, minced
- 3 small yellow onions, sliced
- 3 bell peppers (mixed colors), seeded and thinly sliced
- 4 cups baby arugula or mixed greens

Pat the steaks dry with paper towels. In a small bowl, combine the chipotle powder, ½ teaspoon of the salt, the cumin, and the coriander. Rub the spice mixture all over the steaks and set aside.

In a large cast-iron skillet or heavy sauté pan, heat 1 tablespoon of the olive oil over medium heat until shimmering. Add the garlic and onions and cook, stirring occasionally, until the onions are very soft and light golden brown, 10 to 12 minutes. Add the bell peppers and remaining ½ teaspoon salt and continue to cook until the peppers are very soft, another 8 to 10 minutes.

Line a large serving platter with the arugula. Remove the onions and peppers from the pan and arrange them over the arugula on the platter.

Rinse out the pan, then return it to the stove. Heat the remaining 1 tablespoon olive oil over high heat until shimmering. Place the steaks in the pan.

Cook the steaks for 4 minutes on one side, then flip and cook for another 4 minutes for medium-rare (internal temperature should be

135°F). Remove the steaks from the pan and allow them to rest for 10 minutes on a small rack set over a plate or sheet pan to collect any juices.

Once the steaks have rested, transfer them to a cutting board and slice thinly against the grain. Arrange the sliced steak on top of the peppers on the platter, drizzle any accumulated juices over the meat, and serve.

Nutritional analysis per serving: *Calories: 360, Fat: 16 g, Saturated Fat: 3 g, Cholesterol: 94 mg, Fiber: 4 g, Protein: 42 g, Carbohydrates: 14 g, Sodium: 497 mg*

THE RECIPES

Filet Mignon with Garlic Sauce and Roasted Tomatoes

Serves: 4

Prep Time:
15 minutes

Cook Time:
1 hour and
15 minutes

The roasted tomatoes in this dish are excellent served warm, cold, or at room temperature—which is helpful when you have guests coming for dinner and you don't want to cook while entertaining.

- 4 large heads garlic, unpeeled
- 4½ tablespoons extra-virgin olive oil
- 2 pints cherry or grape tomatoes
- ¾ teaspoon sea salt
- ½ teaspoon freshly ground black pepper
- 2 tablespoons coconut oil
- 4 (1- to 1¼-inch-thick) filets mignons
- 5 to 6 tablespoons low-sodium chicken stock
- 4 to 6 cups baby arugula

Preheat the oven to 400°F.

Cut the top ½ inch or so off each garlic head, just enough to expose the majority of the garlic cloves. Place each head on a large piece of foil. Drizzle ½ tablespoon of the olive oil over each head; wrap the foil around each head to enclose it in its own pouch.

Place the tomatoes on a large rimmed baking sheet. Drizzle with the remaining 2½ tablespoons olive oil and ¼ teaspoon each of the salt and black pepper and toss. Add the garlic pouches on the side of the baking sheet. Place the tomatoes and garlic in the preheated oven.

Roast the tomatoes until they burst and are caramelized, 45 to 60 minutes, making sure to stir midway through. Remove the garlic after about 50 minutes and let it sit until cool enough to handle. Tent the tomatoes with foil to keep warm.

Season the filets with ¼ teaspoon each of the salt and black pepper. In a large cast-iron pan or other oven-safe skillet, heat the coconut oil over high heat until shimmering. Sear the filets until golden brown on each side, about 5 minutes total. Transfer to the oven and cook until the steaks reach the desired internal temperature, about 8 minutes for medium-rare and 10 minutes for medium (a meat thermometer should register 130°F for medium-rare, 140°F for medium, and 160°F for well-done). Remove the filets from the oven, tent with foil, and let rest for at least 5 minutes.

Meanwhile, grip the bottom of each garlic head and squeeze the roasted garlic into the bowl of a food processor. Add the remaining ¼ teaspoon salt and 5 tablespoons chicken stock. Puree until combined, adding another tablespoon of chicken stock if it is too thick. Transfer to a small saucepan and warm over low heat.

Place a filet mignon on each plate, along with some of the roasted tomatoes. Drizzle the warm roasted garlic sauce over the steaks and serve.

Nutritional analysis per serving: *Calories: 490, Fat: 29 g, Saturated Fat: 8 g, Cholesterol: 120 mg, Fiber: 3 g, Protein: 43 g, Carbohydrates: 17 g, Sodium: 473 mg*

RIB-EYE STEAKS WITH GRILLED RADICCHIO

Serves: 4

Prep Time:
10 minutes

Cook Time:
35 minutes

If you want to infuse a little sweetness into this savory meal, a touch of balsamic vinegar will do the trick.

- 2 large heads radicchio, quartered lengthwise
- 4 tablespoons extra-virgin olive oil
- ½ teaspoon sea salt
- 1½ pounds grass-fed boneless rib-eye steaks (2 inches thick)
- 1 pint grape tomatoes, halved
- 3 shallots, thinly sliced
- ¼ cup balsamic vinegar
- grated zest and juice of 1 lemon
- 2 garlic cloves, minced

Preheat the oven to 475°F.

In a large bowl, toss the radicchio with 2 tablespoons of the oil and ¼ teaspoon of the salt.

Heat a well-seasoned oven-safe grill pan or large oven-safe skillet over high heat. Cook 2 radicchio sections at a time, cut-side down, until the outer leaves are dark brown and crisp, 3 to 5 minutes per side. Transfer the radicchio to a cutting board and thinly slice crosswise.

Season the steaks with the remaining ¼ teaspoon salt. Place them in the pan and cook for 3 to 5 minutes per side. Transfer the pan to the oven and continue to cook the steaks for 6 to 8 minutes for medium (internal temperature should reach 140°F). Transfer the steaks to a cutting board to rest for 10 minutes before slicing.

Add the tomatoes, shallots, vinegar, lemon zest, and garlic to the hot pan. Allow the shallots and tomatoes to wilt slightly, 4 to 5 minutes. Remove from the heat and add the lemon juice. Add the radicchio to the pan and toss to combine.

Slice the steaks against the grain and serve over the radicchio salad.

Nutritional analysis per serving: *Calories: 540, Fat: 36 g, Saturated Fat: 13 g, Cholesterol: 116 mg, Fiber: 4 g, Protein: 36 g, Carbohydrates: 20 g, Sodium: 446 mg*

HERB-CRUSTED BEEF TENDERLOIN

Take care not to overcook these steaks, as grass-fed beef tends to be leaner and will yield a tough and chewy steak when overdone.

- 6 garlic cloves, 3 whole and 3 quartered
- 1 tablespoon plus 2 teaspoons extra-virgin olive oil
- 2 pints grape or cherry tomatoes
- 1 fennel bulb, diced
- ½ teaspoon sea salt
- ½ teaspoon dried oregano
- ½ teaspoon dried thyme
- ½ teaspoon dried sage
- ¼ teaspoon finely chopped dried rosemary
- ¼ teaspoon freshly ground black pepper
- 1 tablespoon grapeseed oil
- 4 (6-ounce) grass-fed beef tenderloin steaks
- 1 large bunch asparagus, trimmed

Preheat the oven to 400°F. Place a rimmed baking sheet in the oven to preheat.

Place the 3 whole garlic cloves on a small piece of foil. Drizzle with 1 teaspoon of the olive oil and seal the garlic in the foil. Place the packet on the baking sheet. Remove the garlic after 15 minutes and confirm it is fully roasted—it will smell slightly sweet and feel soft. Set aside to cool. After the garlic has cooled, peel it and reserve.

While the garlic roasts, in a medium bowl, toss the tomatoes, fennel, the 3 quartered garlic cloves, 1 tablespoon of the olive oil, and ¼ teaspoon of the salt. Carefully distribute the vegetables over the preheated baking sheet and roast until the tomatoes are shriveling and beginning to brown, 35 to 40 minutes. When done, remove the vegetables from the baking sheet, place them in a bowl, and lightly crush the tomatoes with a fork.

In a small bowl, combine the whole roasted garlic cloves, oregano, thyme, sage, rosemary, black pepper, and remaining 1 teaspoon olive oil and mash with a fork to make a paste. Set aside.

Heat the grapeseed oil in a heavy cast-iron skillet or oven-safe sauté pan over high heat until shimmering. Place the steaks in the pan, cook for 2 minutes, then flip and cook for another 2 minutes. While the second side cooks, spread 1 teaspoon of the garlic-herb paste over each steak. Transfer the pan to the oven and cook for 5 to 6 minutes for medium-rare (internal temperature 130°F), or 7 to 8 minutes for medium to medium-well (internal temperature 150°F). Allow the steaks to rest for 10 minutes.

While the steak rests, steam the asparagus: Pour 1 cup of water into the bottom of a medium saucepan and bring it to a boil over high heat. Place a steaming rack or basket over the boiling water. Add the asparagus, cover, and steam until bright green and crisp-tender, 1 to 2 minutes. Divide the asparagus among four dinner plates. Top each plate with a steak and garnish with the roasted tomatoes and fennel.

Nutritional analysis per serving: *Calories: 381, Fat: 20 g, Saturated Fat: 7 g, Cholesterol: 85 mg, Fiber: 5 g, Protein: 40 g, Carbohydrates: 15 g, Sodium: 418 mg*

SLOW-COOKED SHORT RIBS WITH CELERY ROOT PUREE

Serves: 6

Prep Time:
30 minutes

Cook Time:
4 hours
(unattended)
plus 1 hour

This is a great weekend meal; there's nothing difficult about it, nothing takes more than a half-hour of attention, and with the slow cooker going, you can come and go while dinner fixes itself. If you'd rather not use a slow cooker, bring the short ribs and other ingredients to a boil in a 5-quart Dutch oven over high heat. Transfer to a 350°F oven and cook until the meat is falling off the bone, about 3 hours.

- 2 pounds bone-in beef short ribs, cut into 2-inch cubes by your butcher
- ½ cup balsamic vinegar
- 7 garlic cloves, 6 thinly sliced and 1 smashed
- 2 jalapeños, seeded and sliced
- 2 tablespoons Dijon mustard
- grated zest of 2 lemons
- 2 teaspoons sea salt
- 3 large red onions, halved
- 1 celery root, peeled and diced
- 1 (13.5-ounce) can unsweetened coconut milk

Preheat the broiler.

Line a rimmed baking sheet with foil and arrange the short ribs, meat-side up, evenly on the sheet. Place the baking sheet about 4 inches under the broiler. Cook, turning the ribs occasionally, until each side is deep brown, 15 to 20 minutes total.

Combine 2 cups of water, the vinegar, sliced garlic, jalapeños, mustard, lemon zest, and 1½ teaspoons of the salt in a 6-quart slow cooker. Add the ribs in an even layer. Cook on high for 4 hours. The meat should be tender when pierced with a fork.

Preheat the oven to 450°F.

With a slotted spoon, transfer the meat from the slow cooker to a plate. Pour the cooking liquid into a gravy strainer to skim off the fat. Do not discard the fat (you should have about ¼ cup).

Add the skimmed cooking liquid to a medium saucepan. Cook over high heat until glossy and thickened and reduced to about 1 cup, 18 to 20 minutes. Remove from the heat. Moisten the short ribs with about ¼ cup of the sauce and set aside the rest to serve with the meal.

Meanwhile, on a large rimmed baking sheet, toss the onions with the reserved fat and the remaining ½ teaspoon salt. Arrange the onions, cut-side down. Roast, without turning, until the onions are browned on the underside, about 15 minutes. Flip and roast until the onions are tender, about 5 minutes more. Tent with foil and set aside.

Combine the celery root, coconut milk, 1 cup of water, and the smashed garlic in a 3-quart saucepan over medium heat. Bring to a boil, reduce the heat to low, and simmer, stirring occasionally, until the celery root is very tender, 25 to 30 minutes.

Strain the celery root, reserving the cooking liquid. Transfer the celery root and about half of the cooking liquid to a blender. Blend with enough liquid to make a smooth puree, but not a sauce, scraping down the sides of the blender bowl frequently. If you have used all of the cooking liquid and your puree is still too thick, add a little water and continue to blend until it reaches the desired consistency. Transfer to a small saucepan and keep warm.

Serve the short ribs with the celery root puree and roasted onions on the side, along with the gravy.

Nutritional analysis per serving: *Calories: 409 Fat: 31 g, Saturated Fat: 15 g, Cholesterol: 57 mg, Fiber: 3 g, Protein: 15 g, Carbohydrates: 18 g, Sodium: 467 mg*

Spice-Rubbed Beef Filet with Braised Green Beans and Mushrooms

Serves: 4

Prep Time: 15 minutes

Cook Time: 30 minutes

Enjoy these filets with a side salad and Roasted Pepper and Red Onion Relish (page 298) for a sweet bite to accompany a savory meal. The leftover smoky-sweet spice rub for the beef can be used for other meats, fish, chicken, or vegetables.

- 1 teaspoon ground turmeric
- 1 teaspoon sweet or smoked paprika
- 1 teaspoon ground coriander
- 1 teaspoon ground cumin
- 1 teaspoon ground ginger
- 1 teaspoon sea salt
- 4 (6-ounce) grass-fed beef tenderloin steaks
- 3 tablespoon extra-virgin olive oil
- 2 shallots, thinly sliced
- 8 ounces mixed mushrooms (such as button, cremini, shiitake, and/or oyster), trimmed and thinly sliced
- 8 ounces green beans, trimmed and halved if large
- 1 cup low-sodium chicken stock
- 2 tablespoons apple cider vinegar

Preheat the oven to 400°F.

In a small bowl, combine the turmeric, paprika, coriander, cumin, ginger, and salt.

Pat the beef dry with paper towels, then sprinkle ¼ teaspoon of the spice rub on each steak and gently rub it all over the meat. Transfer the remaining spice rub to an airtight container and save for another use.

Heat 2 tablespoons of the olive oil in a large cast-iron skillet or other heavy oven-safe sauté pan over high heat until shimmering. Place the steaks in the pan and cook for 1½ minutes, then flip the steaks and cook for another 1½ minutes. Transfer the pan to the oven and cook for 5 to 6 minutes for medium-rare (internal temperature 130°F), or 7 to 8 minutes for medium-well (internal temperature 150°F). Set aside the steaks to rest for 10 minutes before serving.

Wipe out the pan and place it over medium heat. Add the remaining 1 tablespoon olive oil and the shallots. Cook the shallots until they are fragrant and beginning to caramelize, about 3 minutes. Add the mushrooms and cook until they are softened and exuding their juices, 2 to 3 minutes. Add the green beans and cook for another minute.

Turn the heat to low, add the chicken stock and vinegar, and bring to a gentle simmer. Cook until the liquid has reduced by three-quarters and the beans are tender, 5 to 7 minutes.

To serve, distribute the braised beans and mushrooms among four plates and top each with a steak.

Nutritional analysis per serving: *Calories: 330, Fat: 17 g, Saturated Fat: 4 g, Cholesterol: 95 mg, Fiber: 2 g, Protein: 38 g, Carbohydrates: 12 g, Sodium: 532 mg*

BISON STEAKS WITH WILD MUSHROOM SAUCE AND HARICOTS VERTS

Serves: 4

Prep Time: 20 minutes

Cook Time: 25 minutes

Bison tend to be free-range, grass-fed, and wild for most of their life. This means that bison meat has a higher amount of anti-inflammatory omega-3 fatty acids and a better profile of saturated fats. Research shows that grass-fed meat is higher in stearic saturated fatty acids, which are heart-healthy and do not affect cholesterol levels.

- 6 ounces fresh morels
- 4 ounces fresh shiitake mushrooms, stemmed
- 2 large shallots, very thinly sliced
- 8 tablespoons grapeseed oil
- sea salt and freshly ground black pepper
- 1 pound haricots verts, trimmed
- 4 (6-ounce) grass-fed bison rib-eye steaks
- 8 thyme sprigs, plus additional leaves for garnish
- 1 teaspoon fresh lemon juice
- 1 large omega-3 egg yolk

Preheat the oven to 400°F.

Swish the morels in a bowl of warm water to release all grit. Lift them out, and repeat two times. Cut the morels in half lengthwise. Cut the shiitake mushroom caps into pieces about the same size as the morels. Toss with half of the shallots, 2 tablespoons of the oil, and a pinch each of salt and black pepper on a large rimmed baking sheet. Spread in an even layer on one side of the pan.

On the other side of the pan, toss the haricots verts, remaining shallots, 1 tablespoon of the oil, ¼ teaspoon salt, and a pinch of black pepper. Spread in an even layer. Roast until the vegetables are tender, about 20 minutes. Remove from the oven and set aside.

Meanwhile, season the steaks with ½ teaspoon each salt and black pepper. Heat 2 tablespoons of the oil in a large oven-safe skillet over medium-high heat until shimmering. Add the steaks to the pan and cook until well browned on the bottom, 1 to 2 minutes, then turn and cook until the other side is well browned, another 1 to 2 minutes. Scatter the thyme sprigs on top of the meat and transfer to the oven. Cook alongside the vegetables for 5 to 7 minutes for medium-rare (120°F). Discard the thyme sprigs. Transfer the steaks to serving plates and let them rest for 10 minutes.

Meanwhile, in a small saucepan, gently heat the remaining 3 tablespoons oil over low heat. Fill another saucepan with water and bring to a gentle simmer over medium-low heat. Set a medium bowl over the saucepan and in it whisk the lemon juice, egg yolk, 1 teaspoon of warm water, and ¼ teaspoon salt until thickened and warm. Continue whisking while adding the warmed oil from the other saucepan in a slow, steady stream. While still whisking, add ¼ cup of warm water in a slow, steady stream. Whisk until pale yellow, smooth, and creamy. Gently fold in the mushrooms from the baking sheet.

Spoon the mushrooms and sauce over and around the steaks. Place the haricots verts alongside the steaks. Garnish with thyme leaves and serve.

Nutritional analysis per serving: Calories: 480, Fat: 26 g, Saturated Fat: 4 g, Cholesterol: 150 mg, Fiber: 6 g, Protein: 43 g, Carbohydrates: 19 g, Sodium: 518 mg

Mexican "Rice" Bowl

Serves: 4

Prep Time:
20 minutes

Cook Time:
20 minutes

Serve this fun, cheerful dish at your next family gathering to introduce the versatility and flavor that cooking with whole foods affords. This recipe incorporates cauliflower "rice" for a grain-free alternative.

- 1 medium carrot, peeled
- 5 medium radishes
- ½ cucumber
- 2 scallions, chopped
- 1½ to 2 tablespoons cider vinegar
- sea salt and freshly ground black pepper
- 2 tablespoons plus 1 teaspoon coconut oil
- 1 teaspoon minced garlic
- 1 pound grass-fed ground beef
- ½ teaspoon ground cumin
- ¼ teaspoon crushed red pepper flakes
- 1 head cauliflower
- 1 small yellow onion, finely chopped
- 1 avocado, pitted, peeled, and diced, for garnish
- ½ cup chopped fresh cilantro, for garnish
- lime wedges, for serving

Using a box grater, grate the carrot, radishes, and cucumber into a medium bowl. Mix in the scallions, 1½ tablespoons of the vinegar, and ¼ teaspoon each salt and black pepper. Stir to combine; taste, adding ½ tablespoon more vinegar, if desired.

In a medium sauté pan, warm 1 teaspoon of the coconut oil over medium-high heat until shimmering. Add the garlic and cook, stirring constantly, for 30 seconds. Add the ground beef, along with the cumin, red pepper flakes, and ¼ teaspoon salt. Sauté, breaking up the beef with a wooden spoon, until fully cooked, 7 to 8 minutes. Transfer to a dish and tent with foil to keep warm.

Cut the cauliflower in half. Place a box grater over a large bowl and grate each cauliflower half over the big holes of the grater—hold the cauliflower by its stem as you grate it into "rice." Alternatively, you can coarsely chop the core and the florets and pulse them together in a food processor until they are reduced to the size of couscous or rice grains— be careful not to overprocess.

Heat the remaining 2 tablespoons coconut oil in a nonstick pan over medium-high heat until shimmering. Add the onion and cook until softened, 2 to 3 minutes. Add the cauliflower and combine. Cook, stirring frequently, until the cauliflower is slightly crispy on the outside but tender on the inside, 5 to 8 minutes. Season with a pinch of salt.

Divide the cauliflower "rice" among four bowls. Top each with beef and grated vegetables. Garnish with avocado and cilantro and serve with lime wedges.

Nutritional analysis per serving: *Calories: 430, Fat: 30 g, Saturated Fat: 9 g, Cholesterol: 70 mg, Fiber: 8 g, Protein: 27 g, Carbohydrates: 17 g, Sodium: 430 mg*

BEEF BOLOGNESE

Serves: 4

Prep Time:
20 minutes

Cook Time:
1 hour

Try this take on Bolognese—but instead of serving over pasta, substitute low-carb shirataki noodles, which give this dish the traditional look and taste without all the extra carbs. Pair with Braised Broccoli with Tomatoes and Roasted Garlic (page 260).

- 1 tablespoon extra-virgin olive oil
- 1 pound grass-fed ground beef
- 1 medium yellow onion, finely chopped
- 10 ounces button mushrooms, trimmed and sliced
- 1 medium zucchini, grated
- 2 garlic cloves, minced
- 1 (28-ounce) can diced tomatoes
- ¾ teaspoon dried oregano
- ½ teaspoon dried thyme
- ½ teaspoon dried basil
- ½ teaspoon sea salt
- ¼ teaspoon freshly ground black pepper
- 2 bay leaves
- 2 (6- to 8-ounce) bags shirataki noodles, well rinsed
- 2 tablespoons chopped fresh basil, for garnish

In a medium stockpot, warm ½ tablespoon of the oil over medium-high heat until shimmering. Add the ground beef and sauté until it is fully cooked, about 8 minutes. Using a slotted spoon, transfer the meat to a bowl, leaving any oil in the pot.

Add the remaining ½ tablespoon oil to the pot. Add the onion and sauté until softened, about 8 minutes. Add the mushrooms and sauté until softened, 5 to 6 minutes. Stir in the grated zucchini and sauté until wilted, another few minutes.

Add the garlic and cook, stirring, for 30 seconds. Add the chopped tomatoes with their juices, reserved ground beef, dried herbs, salt, black pepper, and bay leaves. Stir to combine. Let the sauce come to a boil and then reduce the heat to a simmer. Cover halfway with a lid and cook for 30 minutes. Remove the bay leaves.

Cook the shirataki noodles in boiling water according to the package directions. Transfer the cooked noodles to a colander. Blot the noodles dry with paper towels.

In a large bowl, toss the noodles with the meat sauce. Garnish with the fresh basil and serve.

Nutritional analysis per serving: *Calories: 322, Fat: 17 g, Saturated Fat: 6 g, Cholesterol: 70 mg, Fiber: 5 g, Protein: 26 g, Carbohydrates: 18 g, Sodium: 397 mg*

SUMMER PESTO "PASTA" WITH GROUND LAMB

Serves: 4

Prep Time:
30 minutes

Cook Time:
15 minutes

Eating the 10-Day Detox way is not about restriction or deprivation—it's about healthful satisfaction. This meal replaces traditional flour-based pasta with zucchini ribbons and features bright pesto flavors, giving you the feeling of a pasta-based meal without all the refined ingredients.

- ½ cup pine nuts
- 2 cups loosely packed fresh basil leaves
- 2 garlic cloves, halved
- 1 teaspoon sea salt
- ½ teaspoon freshly ground black pepper
- 2 tablespoons extra-virgin olive oil
- 5 large zucchini
- 1 pound ground grass-fed lamb
- 2 medium tomatoes, chopped

In the bowl of a food processor, process the pine nuts until finely chopped, about 30 seconds. Add the basil leaves, garlic, and ¼ teaspoon each salt and black pepper and pulse until combined. Drizzle the olive oil and 1 tablespoon of water through the feed tube and continue to puree until a smooth consistency is achieved, scraping down the mixture as needed. Reserve the pesto.

Trim the ends of each zucchini. Using a mandolin (or a vegetable peeler), slice the zucchini lengthwise into thin ribbons. Cut the ribbons in half crosswise so they don't tear while sautéing.

In a large nonstick sauté pan, sauté the lamb and ¼ teaspoon of the salt over medium-high heat until fully cooked, 6 to 8 minutes. Use a slotted spoon to transfer the meat to a bowl, leaving the juices from the lamb in the pan. Tent the meat with foil to keep warm.

Add half of the zucchini ribbons to the drippings in the pan and sauté, stirring constantly, until the zucchini is softened, 3 to 4 minutes. Transfer the zucchini to a large bowl. Repeat with the remaining zucchini ribbons.

Use a paper towel to blot excess moisture from the zucchini and season with the remaining ½ teaspoon salt and ¼ teaspoon black pepper. Top the zucchini with the pesto, lamb, and tomatoes. Using tongs, gently mix the ingredients to combine, and serve.

Nutritional analysis per serving: *Calories: 570, Fat: 44 g, Saturated Fat: 15 g, Cholesterol: 85 mg, Fiber: 7 g, Protein: 26 g, Carbohydrates: 19 g, Sodium: 438 mg*

Lamb and Mustard Green Stir-Fry

Pair this dish with an appetizer like Creamy Herbed Tahini Dip with vegetables (page 281).

(page 281).

Serves: 4

Prep Time:
20 minutes

Cook Time:
10 minutes

- 1 tablespoon cumin seeds
- 1 teaspoon Szechuan or black peppercorns
- ½ teaspoon crushed red pepper flakes
- 2 tablespoons grapeseed oil
- 10 garlic cloves, thinly sliced
- 4 scallions, thinly sliced, white and green parts separated
- 1 (1¼-pound) boneless leg of grass-fed lamb, thinly sliced
- ¾ teaspoon sea salt
- 1 tablespoon gluten-free, low-sodium tamari
- 1 bunch mustard greens, stemmed and chopped
- 1 tablespoon apple cider vinegar
- ½ jalapeño, seeded and very thinly sliced
- ¼ cup chopped fresh cilantro

In a large skillet, heat the cumin seeds and peppercorns over medium heat, tossing occasionally, until toasted, about 2 minutes. Cool, then transfer to a spice grinder, along with the red pepper flakes, and coarsely grind. Set aside.

Heat 1 tablespoon of the oil in the same skillet over medium-high heat until shimmering. Add half of the garlic and half of the scallion whites and cook, stirring, for 30 seconds. Add the lamb, sprinkle with half of the spice mix and ½ teaspoon of the salt, and cook, stirring occasionally, until browned, about 2 minutes. Stir in the tamari and transfer to a plate.

Add the remaining 1 tablespoon oil to the skillet. Add the remaining garlic, scallion whites, and spice mix. Cook, stirring, until just fragrant, about 1 minute. Add the mustard greens and sprinkle with the remaining ¼ teaspoon salt. Cook, stirring, until the greens are just wilted, about 2 minutes. Stir in the vinegar and the lamb with all its accumulated juices.

Transfer to a serving dish. Top with the scallion greens, jalapeño, and cilantro and serve.

Nutritional analysis per serving: Calories: 290, Fat: 13 g, Saturated Fat: 3 g, Cholesterol: 90 mg, Fiber: 4 g, Protein: 33 g, Carbohydrates: 10 g, Sodium: 543 mg

LAMB KORMA

Serves: 6

Prep Time:
15 minutes

Cook Time:
2 hours and
15 minutes

Korma is a dish from northern India, typically made from lamb, cream, and sweet, toasty spices. Coconut milk is a great alternative for the dairy in this version. Adjust the cayenne to suit your heat preference; it's not typically a spicy dish, but feel free to crank up the heat if you like. Korma, like most stews, tastes better after a day or two in the refrigerator. Serve with a side of roasted cauliflower or Swiss chard.

- 2 pounds grass-fed lamb stew meat, cut into 1-inch pieces
- 1 teaspoon sea salt
- 2 tablespoons extra-virgin olive oil
- 1 medium yellow onion, diced
- 8 garlic cloves, minced
- 1 tablespoon minced fresh ginger
- 2 teaspoons ground cumin
- 1 teaspoon ground coriander
- ½ teaspoon ground turmeric
- ½ teaspoon ground cinnamon
- ½ teaspoon cayenne pepper, or to taste
- ¼ teaspoon fennel seeds
- 1 cup canned crushed or diced tomatoes with juices
- 1 (13.5-ounce) can full-fat unsweetened coconut milk
- ½ cup loosely packed chopped fresh cilantro, for garnish

Preheat the oven to 350°F.

Pat the lamb dry with paper towels, then sprinkle with the salt. In a large oven-safe sauté pan or Dutch oven, heat the oil over high heat until shimmering. Working in batches if necessary so as not to crowd the pan, brown the lamb cubes all over, about 30 seconds per side.

Transfer the lamb to a plate and reduce the heat to medium. Add the onion, garlic, and ginger and cook until the onion begins to soften and become fragrant, 2 to 3 minutes, stirring constantly to avoid burning the garlic. Add the cumin, coriander, turmeric, cinnamon, cayenne, and fennel seed and cook until the spices are fragrant, about 1 minute.

Return the lamb and any accumulated juices to the pan, and then add the tomatoes and coconut milk. Stir well, and bring to a simmer.

Cover the pan and transfer it to the oven. Cook for 1½ hours, then uncover the pan and continue to cook until the lamb is fork-tender, about 30 minutes more. If the sauce is getting very thick before the lamb is done, add 1 tablespoon of water at a time to reach the desired consistency.

Serve the lamb stew garnished with the cilantro.

Nutritional analysis per serving: Calories: 429, Fat: 26 g, Saturated Fat: 12 g, Cholesterol: 100 mg, Fiber: 1 g, Protein: 38 g, Carbohydrates: 8 g, Sodium: 491 mg

LEBANESE-STYLE LAMB STEW

The texture and flavor of this hearty stew will keep your mouth happily entertained. Enjoy this robust dish the next time you crave comfort food.

- 2 tablespoons extra-virgin olive oil
- 2½ pounds grass-fed lamb shanks
- sea salt and freshly ground black pepper
- 1 large yellow onion, chopped
- 3 garlic cloves, thinly sliced
- 1 teaspoon ground ginger
- ½ teaspoon ground allspice
- ½ teaspoon ground cloves
- ½ teaspoon ground cinnamon
- ½ teaspoon freshly grated nutmeg
- 1 (28-ounce) can whole tomatoes
- 2 pounds eggplant, trimmed and cut into ¾-inch cubes
- 1 large bunch lacinato kale, tough stems removed, leaves sliced
- grated zest of 1 lemon
- 1 cup chopped fresh parsley
- lemon wedges, for serving

Serves: 4

Prep Time:
20 minutes

Cook Time:
2 hours and
15 minutes

Heat 1 tablespoon of the oil in a large Dutch oven over medium-high heat until shimmering. Season the lamb with ½ teaspoon salt and ¼ teaspoon black pepper and add to the pot. Cook, turning occasionally, until evenly browned, about 5 minutes. Transfer the lamb to a plate. Drain and discard the fat. Carefully wipe the pot clean with paper towels.

Heat the remaining 1 tablespoon oil in the same pot over medium heat. Add the onion and garlic, season with a pinch of salt, and stir well. Add 2 tablespoons of warm water and cook, stirring occasionally, until the onion is brown and crisp-tender, about 5 minutes. Add the ginger, allspice, cloves, cinnamon, and nutmeg. Cook, stirring, for 30 seconds. Add the tomatoes with their juices. Gently smash the tomatoes into small pieces with the back of a spoon. Return the lamb to the pot, nestle the meat in the mixture, and spoon the tomatoes on top. Cover, reduce the heat to low, and simmer for 1½ hours.

Meanwhile, dissolve 1½ teaspoons salt in 5 cups of warm water in a large bowl. Add the eggplant pieces, weigh them down with a 6- to 8-inch plate, and soak for 30 minutes. Drain, rinse, and drain again.

After the lamb has simmered for 1½ hours, transfer the shanks to a plate, leaving the sauce in the pot. Stir the eggplant and kale into the pot. Simmer, uncovered, over low heat, stirring occasionally, until the egg-plant is almost tender, about 20 minutes. When the lamb is cool enough to handle, pull the meat from the bones and discard the bones. Stir the meat into the pot and simmer until the eggplant is tender but still holding its shape, about 10 minutes. Stir in the lemon zest.

Season with ½ teaspoon each salt and black pepper and divide among four serving dishes. Sprinkle the parsley on top and serve with the lemon wedges.

Nutritional analysis per serving: *Calories 440, Fat 17 g, Saturated Fat 4 g, Cholesterol 125 g, Fiber 13 g, Protein 41 g, Carbohydrate 35 g, Sodium 430 mg.*

ROAST PORK TENDERLOIN WITH
COCONUT CURRY VEGETABLES

Serves: 4

Prep Time:
35 minutes

Cook Time:
1 hour

Shop at your local farmers' market during the summer months to procure vegetables at their peak for this dish. Fresh food has more flavor and nutrition—a win–win for your detoxification process. If you like a lot of heat, leave the seeds in the serrano chiles.

- 1 small eggplant, cut into ½-inch cubes
- 4 tablespoons plus 2 teaspoons extra-virgin olive oil
- sea salt
- 1 zucchini, halved lengthwise and cut into ½-inch-thick slices
- 1 yellow summer squash, halved lengthwise and cut into ½-inch-thick slices
- 3 small yellow onions, roughly chopped
- 2 or 3 serrano chiles, seeded and coarsely chopped
- 4 garlic cloves, halved
- 1 (2-inch) piece ginger, peeled and sliced
- 2 teaspoons garam masala
- 1 teaspoon ground turmeric
- ¼ cup coriander seeds
- 3 bay leaves
- 1 cinnamon stick
- 3 black cardamom pods
- 1 teaspoon cumin seeds
- 1 (14.5-ounce) can diced tomatoes
- 1 (5.4-ounce) can unsweetened coconut cream
- juice of 2 lemons
- ½ cup lightly packed chopped fresh cilantro, plus more for garnish
- 1 (1½-pound) pork tenderloin, halved lengthwise
- 2 tablespoons coconut oil
- ½ teaspoon ground cinnamon
- pinch of cayenne pepper

Preheat the oven to 475°F.

Line two rimmed baking sheets with foil. On one sheet, toss the eggplant with 2 tablespoons of the olive oil and ¼ teaspoon salt. On the other sheet, toss the zucchini and summer squash with 2 teaspoons of the olive oil and ¼ teaspoon salt. Roast, tossing occasionally and rotating the sheets halfway through, until the vegetables are tender and beginning to brown, 25 to 30 minutes. When the vegetables are done, preheat the broiler.

Meanwhile, in the bowl of a food processor, process the onions, chiles, garlic, ginger, garam masala, turmeric, and 1¼ teaspoons salt into a thick paste. Set aside.

In an extra-large skillet, combine the coriander seeds, bay leaves, cinnamon stick, cardamom pods, and cumin seeds. Over medium-high heat, cook the spices, stirring often, until fragrant, 2 to 3 minutes. Using a spice grinder (or clean coffee grinder), grind the mixture.

Add the remaining 2 tablespoons olive oil to the skillet and heat over medium heat. Add the ground spice mixture and warm, stirring constantly, until the spices are fragrant, about 1 minute. Add the reserved onion paste and cook, stirring occasionally, until the paste is golden-brown, about 10 minutes.

Add the diced tomatoes with their juices. Continue to cook, stirring occasionally, until the oil begins to separate and the paste becomes thinner and smoother, 10 to 12 minutes. Reserve 2¼ cups of the tomato mixture for the curry sauce and store any extra in a covered glass jar in the refrigerator for up to 3 days.

Add the coconut cream to the tomato mixture and raise the heat to medium-high until you reach a gentle simmer. Stir well.

Add the roasted eggplant, zucchini, and summer squash. Cook until the vegetables have absorbed some of the sauce and are completely tender, 6 to 8 minutes. Stir in the lemon juice and cilantro. Reduce the heat as low as possible and cover to keep warm.

On a rimmed baking sheet lined with foil, brush the pork with the coconut oil, season with the ground cinnamon and cayenne, and sprinkle with a pinch of salt.

Broil the pork about 5 inches from the heat source, turning once, until the pork is fragrant and the spices are beginning to brown, 15 to 20 minutes; an instant-read thermometer inserted into the thickest part should register 160°F.

Slice the pork and divide it among four plates. Serve with some of the curry vegetable sauce.

Nutritional analysis per serving: *Calories: 547, Fat: 36 g, Saturated Fat: 18 g, Cholesterol: 87 mg, Fiber: 11 g, Protein: 315 g, Carbohydrates: 24 g, Sodium: 446 mg*

VEGETABLES AND SIDE DISHES

ARUGULA AND FENNEL SALAD

Serves: 4

Prep Time:
10 minutes

Arugula is one of my favorite greens. Here, the peppery zing of the arugula is matched perfectly with the slightly sweet crunch of the fennel. This salad will nicely complement any chicken, meat, or fish dish.

- 3 tablespoons extra-virgin olive oil
- juice of 1 lemon
- 2 small fennel bulbs, cored and thinly sliced
- 6 ounces baby arugula
- ¼ teaspoon sea salt
- pinch of freshly ground black pepper
- 2 tablespoons toasted pepitas, for garnish

In a large salad bowl, whisk the olive oil and lemon juice until combined. Add the sliced fennel and baby arugula. Season with the salt and black pepper and toss well. Garnish with pepitas and serve.

Nutritional analysis per serving: *Calories: 170, Fat: 14 g, Saturated Fat: 2 g, Cholesterol: 0 mg, Fiber: 5 g, Protein: 4 g, Carbohydrates: 11 g, Sodium: 220 mg*

HEIRLOOM TOMATO, CUCUMBER, AND RADISH SALAD

Serves: 4

Prep Time:
10 minutes

Heirloom tomatoes are old varieties that until recently were not widely grown or sold. Many of these beauties have been resurrected from obscurity and are unique in their colors, shapes, and widely varying flavors. If you can't find heirlooms, just use a mix of different tomatoes—whatever is freshest and ripest at your market. Never store tomatoes in the refrigerator; it destroys their flavor and stops them from further ripening.

- 1 pound mixed heirloom tomatoes, cut into slices, wedges, and/or halves
- 1 small cucumber, thinly sliced
- 2 large radishes, thinly sliced
- 2 tablespoons slivered almonds
- 2 tablespoons extra-virgin olive oil
- ¼ teaspoon sea salt
- pinch of freshly ground black pepper
- 6 large fresh basil or mint leaves, thinly sliced

Arrange the tomatoes, cucumber, and radishes on a serving plate or on four individual plates. Sprinkle the almonds over the vegetables.

Drizzle the olive oil over the salad, then sprinkle with the salt, black pepper, and basil or mint. Serve.

Nutritional analysis per serving: *Calories: 100, Fat: 8 g, Saturated Fat: 1 g, Cholesterol: 0 mg, Fiber: 1 g, Protein: 2 g, Carbohydrates: 6 g, Sodium: 160 mg*

GREEN BEANS AND ALMONDS

Serves: 4

Prep Time:
10 minutes

Cook Time:
5 minutes

Walnut and hazelnut oils are a true treat for your senses—not to mention your body. To maintain the phytonutrients and delicate healthy fats, select unrefined oil and store at room temperature for up to 6 months.

- sea salt and freshly ground black pepper
- 1½ pounds green beans, trimmed and halved
- 2 teaspoons Dijon mustard
- 2 teaspoons apple cider vinegar
- ½ shallot, minced
- 1 garlic clove, minced
- 2 tablespoons extra-virgin olive oil
- 1 tablespoon walnut or hazelnut oil
- ¼ cup slivered almonds

Bring a 5-quart pot of water to a boil over high heat. Add 1 tablespoon salt. Add the green beans and cook until crisp-tender, 3 to 4 minutes. Drain and immediately rinse with cold water.

Whisk together the mustard, vinegar, shallot, and garlic in a small bowl. Whisk in the olive and nut oils until combined. Season with a pinch each of salt and black pepper.

Drain the cooled beans and pat them dry, then transfer them to a serving bowl. Toss the beans with the dressing, and then gently mix in the almonds. Serve.

Nutritional analysis per serving: *Calories: 163, Fat: 10 g, Saturated Fat: 1 g, Cholesterol: 0 mg, Fiber: 6 g, Protein: 5 g, Carbohydrates: 17 g, Sodium: 185 mg*

SHREDDED BRUSSELS SPROUTS WITH
WARM WALNUT DRESSING

Serves: 4

Prep Time:
15 minutes

Cook Time:
5 minutes

Warming the dressing for this salad brings out the flavor of the mustard seeds and takes the raw edge off the shallot and garlic. It will also slightly wilt the shredded Brussels sprouts, allowing them to soak up the flavors and tenderize. Best of all, this salad can be served warm, at room temperature, or chilled.

- 1 pound Brussels sprouts, shredded
- 2 tablespoons grapeseed oil
- 2 tablespoons extra-virgin olive oil
- 1 tablespoon minced shallot
- 1 garlic clove, minced
- 1 teaspoon brown or black mustard seeds (if you can't find either, yellow is fine)
- 2 tablespoons apple cider vinegar
- ¼ teaspoon sea salt
- pinch of freshly ground black pepper
- ¼ cup chopped walnuts
- 1 tablespoon minced fresh chives, for garnish (optional)

Pour 1 cup of water into the bottom of a medium saucepan and bring it to a boil over high heat. Place a steaming rack or basket over the boiling water. Add the Brussels sprouts, cover, and steam until tender, 3 to 5 minutes. Transfer to a large bowl and allow them to cool.

In a small skillet, heat both of the oils over low heat. Add the shallot, garlic, mustard seeds, vinegar, salt, and black pepper. When the dressing is slightly warm, drizzle it over the Brussels sprouts. Mix to coat evenly. Top with the walnuts and chives, if desired.

Nutritional analysis per serving: *Calories: 217, Fat: 19 g, Saturated Fat: 2 g, Cholesterol: 0 mg, Fiber: 4 g, Protein: 5 g, Carbohydrates: 11 g, Sodium: 168 mg*

SWISS CHARD WITH PINE NUTS AND SCALLIONS

Serves: 4

Prep Time:
15 minutes

Cook Time:
5 minutes

Chard and other leafy greens make great side dishes or bases for cooked vegetable salads. Chop up any leftover vegetables you have and serve them over sautéed greens, with a tasty vinaigrette. Add a poached or hard-boiled egg, some grilled fish, or a can of sardines for a complete meal.

- 2 tablespoons extra-virgin olive oil
- 3 garlic cloves, minced
- 1 large bunch Swiss chard, cut into ½-inch-wide strips
- 2 scallions, thinly sliced
- 2 tablespoons pine nuts
- 2 teaspoons fresh lemon juice
- ½ teaspoon sea salt
- ¼ cup thinly sliced basil, for garnish (optional)

Heat a large sauté pan over medium heat until shimmering. Add the olive oil and garlic and cook for 1 minute.

Add the chard to the pan, increase the heat to high, and toss the chard to distribute the oil and garlic evenly. Cover the pan and cook for 1 minute.

Uncover the pan and continue to cook, stirring, until the chard is totally wilted and the juices in the pan fully evaporate, 3 to 4 minutes.

Scatter the scallions and pine nuts over the chard, and sprinkle with lemon juice and salt. Serve garnished with basil, if desired.

Nutritional analysis per serving: *Calories: 113, Fat: 10 g, Saturated Fat: 1 g, Cholesterol: 0 mg, Fiber: 2 g, Protein: 3 g, Carbohydrates: 6 g, Sodium: 395 mg*

WILTED MIZUNA WITH WALNUTS

Serves: 4

Prep Time:
5 minutes

Cook Time:
20 minutes

Inspired by the flavors frequently found in southern Indian cooking, this recipe highlights the sweetness of toasted coconut contrasted with the spicy greens.

- sea salt
- 12 ounces green beans, trimmed
- ¼ cup unsweetened coconut flakes
- 3 tablespoons chopped walnuts
- 1 tablespoon coconut oil
- 1 tablespoon cumin seeds
- 1 tablespoon black or yellow mustard seeds
- 2 medium yellow onions, finely chopped
- 1 tablespoon apple cider vinegar
- 12 ounces mizuna or arugula

Bring a large saucepan of water to a boil over high heat. Add 1 teaspoon salt. Add the green beans and cook just until they are crisp-tender, about 4 minutes. Drain.

Meanwhile, toast the coconut flakes and walnuts in a large skillet over medium heat, tossing occasionally, until golden brown and fragrant, about 5 minutes. Transfer to a plate and reserve.

Heat the oil in the same skillet over medium heat. Add the cumin and mustard seeds and cook, stirring, until the seeds are fragrant and begin to pop, about 20 seconds. Add the onions and a pinch of salt and cook, stirring occasionally, until translucent and tender, about 7 minutes. Add the vinegar and cook until it has evaporated.

Add half of the mizuna and ¼ teaspoon salt. Cook, stirring, until wilted, about 2 minutes. Add the remaining mizuna, the green beans, and ¼ teaspoon salt. Fold gently until all of the mizuna is wilted. Transfer to a serving dish and top with the toasted walnuts and coconut flakes. Serve.

Nutritional analysis per serving: *Calories: 171, Fat: 12 g, Saturated Fat: 6 g, Cholesterol: 0 mg, Fiber 7 g, Protein: 6 g, Carbohydrates: 15 g, Sodium: 421 mg*

WILD MUSHROOM SAUTÉ

Serves: 4

Prep Time:
15 minutes

Cook Time:
10 minutes

A simple yet delicious side with robust flavors—perfect over shirataki noodles or your favorite steamed vegetables.

- 2 tablespoons extra-virgin olive oil
- 1 large shallot, finely chopped
- ¾ teaspoon sea salt
- 10 ounces maitake or shiitake mushrooms, trimmed and cut into ½-inch pieces
- 8 ounces oyster mushrooms, trimmed and cut into ½-inch pieces
- 5 ounces cremini mushrooms, trimmed and cut into ½-inch pieces
- ¼ teaspoon freshly ground black pepper
- 1 teaspoon toasted sesame seeds
- grated zest and juice of 1 lime

Heat the oil in a large skillet over medium-high heat until shimmering. Add the shallot and ¼ teaspoon of the salt. Cook until lightly browned, about 1 minute, stirring constantly.

Add the mushrooms, the remaining ½ teaspoon salt, and the black pepper. Cook until the mushrooms are brown and tender, about 8 minutes, stirring occasionally. The natural juices from the mushrooms will release and then evaporate.

Transfer the mushrooms to a serving platter and sprinkle with the sesame seeds, lime zest, and lime juice. Serve.

Nutritional analysis per serving: *Calories: 120, Fat: 8 g, Saturated Fat: 1 g, Cholesterol: 0 mg, Fiber: 4 g, Protein: 4 g, Carbohydrates: 12 g, Sodium: 418 mg*

Spicy Cauliflower Sauté

Serves: 4

Prep Time:
10 minutes

Cook Time:
40 minutes

This side dish is so packed with flavor it will make a believer out of anyone who says vegetables are boring. Enjoy as a side dish or even as a snack or hors d'oeuvre at your next social gathering.

- 4 tablespoons grapeseed oil
- 1 head cauliflower, cored, florets cut into bite-size pieces
- 1 red bell pepper, seeded and sliced into ½-inch strips
- 2 jalapeños, seeded and thinly sliced
- 3 garlic cloves, minced
- 1 tablespoon gluten-free, low-sodium tamari
- lime wedges, for serving

In a large sauté pan, warm 2 tablespoons of the oil and ⅔ cup of water over medium–high heat. Add half of the cauliflower and allow it to cook, stirring occasionally. After the water begins to evaporate and the cauliflower starts to fry in the oil, continue to stir until the cauliflower is brown and crisp, 6 to 8 minutes. Using a slotted spoon, transfer the cauliflower to a plate.

Cook the remaining cauliflower in the same way. During the last 2 minutes of cooking, add the bell pepper, jalapeños, and garlic. Then return the first batch of cauliflower to the pan, add the tamari, and toss to combine.

Serve with lime wedges.

Nutritional analysis per serving: *Calories: 210 Fat: 15 g, Saturated Fat: 1.5 g, Cholesterol: 0 mg, Fiber: 7 g, Protein: 6 g, Carbohydrates: 18 g, Sodium: 260 mg*

Braised Broccoli with Tomatoes and Roasted Garlic

Serves: 4

Prep Time:
10 minutes

Cook Time:
15 minutes

Serving whole broccoli spears makes for a creative way to enjoy a whole head of broccoli. To make spears, separate the crown from the stem (both sections should be about the same length). Peel off the tough outer skin of the stem and cut lengthwise into ½-inch-thick strips. Cut the crown (the florets) into long spears with ½-inch-wide stems.

- 2 tablespoons extra-virgin olive oil
- ½ cup thinly sliced red onion
- 1 large head broccoli, cut into spears (see headnote)
- 2 tablespoons mashed Roasted Garlic with Olive Oil and Rosemary (page 287)
- ½ cup low-sodium chicken stock
- 1 cup diced tomatoes
- 1 tablespoon minced fresh rosemary or ½ teaspoon dried rosemary
- ½ teaspoon sea salt
- pinch of freshly ground black pepper
- finely shredded fresh basil, for garnish (optional)

Heat the olive oil in a large sauté pan over medium heat until shimmering. Add the red onion and sauté until soft and beginning to brown, 3 to 5 minutes.

Add the broccoli and garlic paste and sauté for another minute, stirring to distribute the garlic throughout the broccoli.

Add the chicken stock, tomatoes, rosemary, salt, and black pepper and bring to a simmer. Reduce the heat to a low simmer, cover the pan, and cook for 5 minutes.

Uncover the pan, give the broccoli a good stir, and continue to cook, uncovered and stirring occasionally, until the liquid has mostly evaporated and the broccoli is quite soft, about 5 minutes. Garnish with basil, if desired, and serve.

Nutritional analysis per serving: *Calories: 120, Fat: 9 g, Saturated Fat: 1 g, Cholesterol: 5 mg, Fiber: 3 g, Protein: 3 g, Carbohydrates: 10 g, Sodium: 340 mg*

GARLIC AND CHILE BROCCOLINI WITH SOFT-BOILED EGGS

Serves: 4

Prep Time:
25 minutes

Cook Time:
7 minutes

Use any leftover broccolini in tomorrow's breakfast. Simply poach or boil an additional egg for more protein, sprinkle on a few chopped nuts for a little crunch, and serve with a side of berries.

- 3 bunches broccolini
- 4 garlic cloves, peeled
- 4 large omega-3 eggs
- 2 tablespoons extra-virgin olive oil
- ¾ tablespoon balsamic vinegar
- ¼ teaspoon crushed red pepper flakes
- ¼ teaspoon sea salt
- pinch of freshly ground black pepper

Bring a large pot of water to a boil over high heat.

While waiting for the water to boil, prepare the broccolini by trimming and discarding the bottom inch of each stalk. Cut the stalks into 2-inch pieces, cutting thicker stalks in half lengthwise. Cut the broccolini florets into bite-size pieces.

When the water is boiling, add the broccolini stalks and garlic. Cook for 3 minutes. Add the florets, and cook for 1 minute. Transfer to a colander to drain, and run cold water over the broccolini and garlic to stop the cooking process.

To soft-boil the eggs, place them in a large saucepan and add enough cold water to cover by 1 inch. Bring to a boil over medium heat; then remove from the heat and cover. Let stand for 2 minutes. Transfer to a bowl with a slotted spoon and cover with cold water.

Remove the cooked garlic from the broccolini. Roughly chop the garlic and then mash it with a fork or the back of a knife. In a large bowl, combine the mashed garlic, olive oil, vinegar, red pepper flakes, salt, and black pepper.

Blot the broccolini with paper towels to remove any excess water. Add to the bowl with the dressing and toss to combine. Divide the broccolini among four plates. Carefully peel each egg and place on top of the broccolini. Serve.

Nutritional analysis per serving: Calories: 162, Fat: 12 g, Saturated Fat: 2 g, Cholesterol: 180 mg, Fiber: 3 g, Protein: 9 g, Carbohydrates: 7 g, Sodium: 234 mg

Broccoli Rabe with Hot Italian Sausage

Serves: 4

Prep Time:
10 minutes

Cook Time:
10 minutes

This dish is delicious served hot or cold, and may be enjoyed as a hearty snack, too. With a fried egg, it makes a great breakfast.

- ¾ teaspoon sea salt
- 1½ pounds broccoli rabe, trimmed of thick stems
- 2 tablespoons grapeseed oil
- 4 garlic cloves, thinly sliced
- 8 ounces hot Italian sausage, casings removed
- grated zest and juice of 1 lemon
- lemon wedges, for serving

Bring a 3-quart saucepan of water to a boil over high heat. Prepare an ice bath by placing 6 ice cubes in a bowl and filling it to the top with cold water; set aside. Add ½ teaspoon salt and the broccoli rabe to the boiling water. Cook until just tender, 1 to 2 minutes. Drain, and transfer to the ice bath. When the broccoli has cooled, drain again and set aside.

Heat the oil in a large skillet over high heat until shimmering. Add the garlic and cook, stirring constantly, until golden, about 20 seconds. Transfer the garlic to a plate and reserve. Add the sausage to the pan and sauté, breaking it up with the back of a spoon. Cook the sausage until it begins to brown and crisp, 3 to 4 minutes.

Add the broccoli rabe, lemon zest, and reserved garlic to the pan. Toss until warmed, 2 to 3 minutes, and season with the remaining ¼ teaspoon salt.

Transfer to a serving plate and sprinkle with the lemon juice. Serve immediately, with additional lemon wedges.

Nutritional analysis per serving: *Calories: 300, Fat: 25 g, Saturated Fat: 7 g, Cholesterol: 45 mg, Fiber: 4 g, Protein: 14 g, Carbohydrates: 7 g, Sodium: 495 mg*

CAULIFLOWER "RICE"

Makes: about
2 cups

Prep Time:
5 minutes

Cook Time:
10 minutes

This recipe is destined to become a family staple. You can adapt it to fit your taste preferences by changing up the seasonings and offering it with a variety of meals.

- 1 head cauliflower
- 2 tablespoons extra-virgin olive oil or coconut oil
- 1 small yellow onion, finely chopped
- pinch of sea salt
- juice of ½ lime (optional)
- pinch of cumin (optional)
- 1 tablespoon chopped fresh cilantro (optional)

Cut the cauliflower in half. Place a box grater over a large bowl and grate each cauliflower half over the big holes of the grater—hold the cauliflower by its stem as you grate it into "rice." Alternatively, you can coarsely chop the core and the florets and pulse them together in a food processor until they are reduced to the size of couscous or rice grains—be careful not to overprocess.

Heat the olive oil in a medium nonstick pan over medium-high heat until shimmering. Add the onion and cook until softened, 2 to 3 minutes.

Add the cauliflower "rice" to the pan and stir to combine. Cook, stirring frequently, until the cauliflower is slightly crispy on the outside but tender on the inside, 5 to 8 minutes. To enhance the flavor, add the lime juice, cumin, and/or cilantro and serve.

Nutritional analysis per serving (½ cup): *Calories: 84, Fat: 8 g, Saturated Fat: 1 g, Cholesterol: 0 mg, Fiber: 2 g, Protein: 1 g, Carbohydrates: 5 g, Sodium: 79 mg*

MASHED CAULIFLOWER WITH HORSERADISH

Serves: 4

Prep Time:
15 minutes

Cook Time:
20 minutes

It may be hard to believe that a rock-hard vegetable can be transformed into a soft, indulgent, and luscious treat, but this cauliflower preparation yields a texture reminiscent of the beloved mashed potato. This dish spares you the blood sugar spikes, though, and leaves you energized. Vidalia onions lend a mellow, sweeter flavor than other onions, but if you can't find them at your market, just substitute 1 medium yellow onion.

- 2 tablespoons grapeseed oil
- ½ large Vidalia onion, finely chopped
- 1½ teaspoons sea salt
- 2 tablespoons pine nuts
- ½ teaspoon freshly grated nutmeg
- 1 head cauliflower, stem trimmed and cut into 1-inch pieces
- 1 tablespoon freshly grated horseradish
- ¼ teaspoon freshly ground black pepper
- 1 tablespoon minced fresh chives

Heat the oil in a small saucepan over medium-low heat. Add the onion and ¼ teaspoon of the salt and cook, stirring occasionally, until the onion is very tender but not browned, about 20 minutes. Stir in the pine nuts and nutmeg and cook for 1 more minute, stirring continuously to avoid burning the nuts.

Meanwhile, bring a large pot of water to a boil over high heat. Add 1 teaspoon of the salt. Cook the cauliflower until it is very tender, about 10 minutes. Drain and transfer to a food processor. Pulse until chopped.

Add the onion mixture to the food processor, along with the horseradish, black pepper, and remaining ¼ teaspoon salt. Pulse until almost completely smooth.

Transfer to a serving bowl, top with the chives, and serve.

Nutritional analysis per serving: *Calories: 200, Fat: 11 g, Saturated Fat: 1 g, Cholesterol: 0 mg, Fiber: 8 g, Protein: 7 g, Carbohydrates: 24 g, Sodium: 430 mg*

SPICY GARLIC EGGPLANT WITH MINT

Serves: 4

Prep Time:
15 minutes

Cook Time:
15 minutes

I love the combination of spicy red pepper flakes and mint. Here, they balance each other beautifully with the neutral eggplant serving as the canvas to carry the flavors. Mint soothes the belly, so for those of you concerned about the spice in this dish, try it with a little extra mint.

- 1½ tablespoons coconut oil
- 2 medium eggplants, diced
- ½ teaspoon sea salt
- ¼ teaspoon freshly ground black pepper
- 3 garlic cloves, minced
- ½ teaspoon crushed red pepper flakes
- 10 fresh mint leaves, julienned, for garnish

In a large nonstick sauté pan or skillet, heat 1 tablespoon of the oil over medium-high heat until shimmering. Add as much eggplant as you can fit in the pan, probably about two-thirds of it, and cook for 3 to 4 minutes, stirring constantly. As the eggplant shrinks a bit, stir in the remaining eggplant, along with the salt and black pepper. Continue sautéing and stirring until the eggplant is tender, 6 to 7 more minutes.

Next, push a bit of eggplant to the side of the pan. Add the remaining ½ tablespoon oil, along with the garlic and red pepper flakes. Stir until the garlic is cooked, 30 seconds to 1 minute. Then, stir to combine with the eggplant. Garnish the eggplant with mint and serve.

Nutritional analysis per serving: Calories: 120, Fat: 6 g, Saturated Fat: 4.5 g, Cholesterol: 0 mg, Fiber: 8 g, Protein: 3 g, Carbohydrates: 17 g, Sodium: 300 mg

STEAMED VEGETABLES WITH LEMON AIOLI

Serves: 8

Prep Time:
15 minutes

Cook Time:
10 minutes

Making aioli is very rewarding, as you transform simple ingredients into a new, unrecognizable form. Keep some around in your refrigerator and dollop on poached eggs for a nice breakfast treat.

- 1 large omega-3 egg yolk
- grated zest of ½ lemon
- 1 garlic clove, halved
- ¼ teaspoon sea salt
- ½ cup extra-virgin olive oil
- 1 pound asparagus, trimmed
- 8 ounces snow peas, trimmed
- 1 large yellow summer squash, cut into ½-inch-thick spears
- 1 red bell pepper, seeded and cut into ¼-inch-thick strips

Combine the egg yolk, lemon zest, garlic, salt, and 1 teaspoon of water in the bowl of a food processor. Pulse a few times; then, with the machine running, stream the oil in through the feed tube and blend until all of the oil is incorporated and the aioli is smooth. Transfer to a small bowl.

Pour 1 cup of water into the bottom of a medium saucepan and bring it to a boil over high heat. Place a steaming rack or basket over the boiling water. Add the asparagus, cover, and steam until bright green and crisp-tender, about 4 minutes. Transfer the asparagus to a platter large enough for all of the vegetables, but keep the water boiling. Steam the snow peas until bright green and crisp-tender, about 2 minutes. Transfer to the platter. Steam the squash until crisp-tender, about 3 minutes. Transfer to the platter.

Add the bell pepper strips to the platter of steamed vegetables and serve with the aioli on the side, for dipping.

Nutritional analysis per serving: *Calories: 150, Fat: 15 g, Saturated Fat: 2 g, Cholesterol: 28 mg, Fiber: 3 g, Protein: 4 g, Carbohydrates: 17 g, Sodium: 87 mg*

ZUCCHINI RIBBONS WITH PEARL ONIONS AND CARDAMOM

Serves: 4

Prep Time:
10 minutes

Cook Time:
15 minutes

Pearl onions are sweet and mild. They're usually sold unpeeled, but some stores now carry them peeled, which makes this dish even faster and easier to prepare (you can just skip the blanching step). This side dish can be served hot, at room temperature, or chilled—making it a versatile addition to your bag of culinary tricks.

- 10 pearl onions
- 2 tablespoons extra-virgin olive oil
- 1 small shallot, thinly sliced
- 1 teaspoon minced fresh ginger
- ½ cup low-sodium chicken stock
- ½ teaspoon sea salt
- 1 zucchini, shaved (with a mandolin or vegetable peeler) into long ribbons
- 2 tablespoons slivered almonds or chopped hazelnuts
- 1 tablespoon julienned fresh mint leaves
- ¼ teaspoon ground cardamom

Bring a large pot of water to a boil over high heat. Prepare an ice bath by placing 6 ice cubes in a bowl and filling it to the top with cold water; set aside. Blanch the onions in the boiling water for 1 to 2 minutes. Remove them from the water and transfer them to the ice bath. Drain them after a couple of minutes, and then you should be able to easily remove the skins.

Heat the olive oil in a large sauté pan over medium heat until shimmering. Add the shallot and sauté gently until soft and beginning to brown, about 2 minutes. Add the ginger and pearl onions and sauté until the onions begin to brown slightly, about 5 minutes.

Add the chicken stock and salt and bring to a gentle simmer, cover the pan, and cook until the stock has completely evaporated, about 5 minutes. Remove the pan from the heat.

Add the zucchini, almonds, mint, and cardamom and toss well to combine and to allow the zucchini to wilt from the residual heat in the pan. Serve.

Nutritional analysis per serving: *Calories: 118, Fat: 9 g, Saturated Fat: 1 g, Cholesterol: 0 mg, Fiber: 2 g, Protein: 2 g, Carbohydrates: 10 g, Sodium: 306 mg*

Braised Celery Hearts in Walnut Oil

Serves: 4

Prep Time:
5 minutes

Cook Time:
25 minutes

While it's great to have a variety of oils to cook with, for this recipe it is fine to substitute another nut oil or additional extra-virgin olive oil if you don't happen to have walnut oil on hand.

- 1 pound organic celery
- 2 tablespoons extra-virgin olive oil
- 1 garlic clove, minced
- 1 bay leaf
- ¼ teaspoon sea salt
- pinch of freshly ground black pepper
- 1 tablespoon walnut oil

Use a vegetable peeler to peel the outer skin off the celery ribs. Trim both ends and cut the hearts in half crosswise.

Warm the olive oil in a large skillet over medium heat until shimmering. Add the celery and cook, turning occasionally, until golden brown on all sides, 8 to 10 minutes. Add 1 cup of water, the garlic, bay leaf, salt, and black pepper. Cover and cook until most of the liquid has evaporated and the celery is tender, 14 to 15 minutes.

Discard the bay leaf and serve the celery drizzled with the walnut oil.

Nutritional analysis per serving: Calories: 110, Fat: 10 g, Saturated Fat: 1.5 g, Cholesterol: 0 mg, Fiber: 2 g, Protein: 0 g, Carbohydrates: 4 g, Sodium: 270 mg

JICAMA FRIES

Serves: 4

Prep Time:
10 minutes

Cook Time:
35 minutes

Jicama is a nonstarchy root vegetable commonly used in Mexico and Southeast Asia. It has a crisp, juicy texture and a slightly sweet flavor. Use it raw in salads and slaws, or cooked in place of starchier root vegetables.

- 1 large jicama, peeled and cut into ¼-inch sticks
- 1 tablespoon extra-virgin olive oil
- ¼ teaspoon sea salt
- pinch of freshly ground black pepper
- ¼ teaspoon smoked or sweet paprika (optional)
- ¼ teaspoon ground cumin (optional)

Preheat the oven to 400°F. Place a large rimmed baking sheet in the oven to preheat.

In a bowl, toss the jicama fries with the olive oil, salt, black pepper, and spices, if desired.

Carefully spread the jicama fries onto the hot baking sheet in a single layer. Roast for 20 minutes; then, give them a stir and roast for another 15 minutes. Serve hot.

Nutritional analysis per serving: *Calories: 145, Fat: 4 g, Saturated Fat: 1 g, Cholesterol: 0 mg, Fiber: 15 g, Protein: 2 g, Carbohydrates: 27 g, Sodium: 157 mg*

SNACKS

CUCUMBER-KALE SMOOTHIE

Serves: 1

Prep Time:
10 minutes

Enjoy this smoothie as a refreshing afternoon pick-me-up to keep you energized and focused. Having a small protein-based snack between 2 p.m. and 4 p.m. helps regulate blood sugar levels and the hormones that keep your body's circadian clock in a comfortable rhythm.

- 1 (4-inch) piece hothouse or English cucumber, peeled
- ¼ cup tightly packed kale leaves
- 2 raw walnuts
- 1 (1-inch) piece ginger, peeled and coarsely chopped
- 2 tablespoons almond butter
- ¾ cup unsweetened almond milk
- 1 tablespoon fresh lemon juice
- 1 tablespoon chia seeds
- 2 large ice cubes

Combine all of the ingredients in a blender and blend on high speed until smooth, 1 to 2 minutes. If the smoothie is too thick, add a little water and blend again until it reaches the desired consistency. Drink immediately.

Nutritional analysis per serving: Calories: 376, Fat: 30 g, Saturated Fat: 4 g, Cholesterol: 0 mg, Fiber: 9 g, Protein: 14 g, Carbohydrates: 17 g, Sodium: 148 mg

Spicy Mocktail

Serves: 1

Prep Time:
20 minutes

This is the spicy afternoon counterpart to your morning vegetable smoothie, with a touch of tofu for added protein.

- ½ cup tightly packed spinach leaves
- ½ tomato, chopped
- 2 celery ribs
- 3 radishes, chopped
- 4 ounces non-GMO silken or soft tofu
- 1 teaspoon fresh lemon juice
- pinch of cayenne pepper, or to taste
- pinch of freshly ground black pepper
- pinch of celery salt
- 2 ice cubes

Place all of the ingredients, except for one celery rib, in a blender and puree until blended, 30 seconds to 1 minute, stopping to scrape down the blender if necessary. Taste and adjust the seasonings as desired.

Pour into a glass. Garnish with the celery stalk and serve.

Nutritional analysis per serving: *Calories: 95, Fat: 4 g, Saturated Fat: 1 g, Cholesterol: 0 mg, Fiber: 4 g, Protein: 7 g, Carbohydrates: 9 g, Sodium: 248 mg*

DEVILED EGGS

Serves: 4

Prep Time:
20 minutes

Cook Time:
5 minutes

Dress up your normal hard-boiled version with this creative twist on deviled eggs. The incredible egg is a power food because it contains phytonutrients, complete protein, and healthy fats. It makes for an ideal low-glycemic afternoon snack.

- 1 small yellow summer squash, coarsely grated
- ½ teaspoon sea salt
- 4 large omega-3 eggs
- 1 scallion, finely chopped
- 2 tablespoons tahini
- 1 tablespoon Mayonnaise (page 299) or Vegenaise
- 2 teaspoons fresh lemon juice
- sesame seeds, for garnish
- cayenne pepper, or smoked or sweet paprika, for garnish

Place the squash in a colander, sprinkle with ¼ teaspoon of the salt, and set the colander in the sink to drain the excess liquid.

Put the eggs in a large saucepan and add enough cold water to cover by 1 inch. Bring to a boil over medium-high heat, remove from the heat, and cover. Let stand for 12 minutes. Transfer the eggs to a bowl with a slotted spoon and cover with cold water. When cold, peel the eggs and cut each in half lengthwise. Scoop out the yolks and place them in a small bowl.

Squeeze as much liquid as possible out of the squash. Add the squash, scallion (reserving some of the greens for garnish), tahini, mayonnaise, and lemon juice to the bowl with the egg yolks. Mix until well combined and season with the remaining ¼ teaspoon salt.

Divide the yolk mixture among the egg white halves. Sprinkle the tops with the reserved scallion greens, sesame seeds, and cayenne pepper, and serve.

Nutritional analysis per serving: *Calories 133, Fat 10 g, Saturated Fat 2 g, Cholesterol 226 mg, Fiber 1 g, Protein 9 g, Carbohydrates 5 g, Sodium 383 mg*

EGG SALAD IN ENDIVE SPEARS

Serves: 4

Prep Time:
15 minutes

Cook Time:
5 minutes

Endive is a slightly bitter vegetable that looks like a small, elongated, pale yellow-green lettuce. The individual leaves are great for holding dips, spreads, and salads. If endive isn't available, you can also use the smaller inner leaves of romaine lettuce, or scoop the egg salad onto cucumber rounds.

- 2 large omega-3 eggs
- 1 celery rib, including leaves, finely diced
- 1 scallion, finely sliced
- 1 tablespoon minced fresh chives, basil, or parsley
- 2 tablespoons Mayonnaise (page 299) or Vegenaise
- 2 teaspoons Dijon or grainy French mustard
- ½ teaspoon ground turmeric
- ¼ teaspoon smoked or sweet paprika
- sea salt and freshly ground black pepper
- 1 Belgian endive, leaves separated

Put the eggs in a large saucepan and add enough cold water to cover by 1 inch. Bring to a boil over medium-high heat, remove from the heat, and cover. Let stand for 12 minutes. Transfer to a bowl with a slotted spoon and cover with cold water. When cold, peel the eggs and dice.

In a small bowl, combine the diced eggs, celery, scallion, and chives and mix gently with a fork. Add the mayonnaise, mustard, turmeric, and paprika and combine. Season with salt and black pepper to taste.

Scoop the egg salad onto the endive leaves and serve.

Nutritional analysis per serving: *Calories: 90, Fat: 8 g, Saturated Fat: 1.5 g, Cholesterol: 95 mg, Fiber: 1 g, Protein: 3 g, Carbohydrates: 2 g, Sodium: 290 mg*

Stuffed Campari Tomatoes

Serves: 4

Prep Time:
20 minutes

Cook Time:
5 minutes

I love growing tomatoes in my summer garden. There is nothing better than inviting a group of friends over to enjoy a bike ride and an afternoon snack featuring homegrown vegetables. You don't have to have a garden to enjoy this recipe with your friends—you just have to appreciate delicious, easy, and satisfying snack foods.

- 2 poblano peppers
- 8 Campari tomatoes
- 1 avocado, peeled and pitted
- ½ bunch cilantro, including stems
- 1½ teaspoons fresh lime juice
- ½ teaspoon sea salt
- 2 tablespoons toasted sunflower seeds

Rest the peppers on the grate of a gas stove. Turn the fire to medium and char the peppers, turning them with tongs, until evenly blackened and blistered, about 5 minutes. (Alternatively, you can roast the peppers over a gas grill or under the broiler.) Transfer to a bowl, cover with plastic wrap, and let steam. When cool enough to handle, rub off the charred skin and discard, along with the stems and seeds.

While the peppers cool, slice off a little from the top and bottom of each tomato to create flat surfaces. Cut the tomatoes in half. Scoop out and discard the seeds.

Transfer the peppers to a food processor, along with the avocado, cilantro, lime juice, and salt. Puree until very smooth. Transfer to a zipper-top plastic bag and snip a hole in one corner. Pipe the avocado mixture into the tomato halves. Top with the sunflower seeds and serve.

Nutritional analysis per serving: Calories: 140, Fat: 9 g, Saturated Fat: 1.5 g, Cholesterol: 0 mg, Fiber: 4 g, Protein: 2 g, Carbohydrates: 12 g, Sodium: 300 mg

BELL PEPPER MINI QUICHES

Serves: 12

Prep Time:
10 minutes

Cook Time:
20 minutes

I make a double batch of these quiches and freeze half. That way, on busy mornings when I am catching a plane or need a snack between meetings, I can pop one in my toaster oven and avoid craving something sweet.

- 1 tablespoon grapeseed oil
- 8 large omega-3 eggs
- 4 bell peppers (yellow, green, and red), seeded and finely chopped
- 1 teaspoon sea salt
- ½ teaspoon cumin
- ¼ teaspoon freshly ground black pepper
- pinch of cayenne pepper, or to taste

Preheat the oven to 450°F. Brush a 12-cup muffin tin with the grapeseed oil.

Whisk the eggs in a large bowl. Add the bell peppers, salt, cumin, black pepper, and cayenne and stir to combine. Divide the egg mixture among the muffin cups, filling them just below the rim. Place the muffin tin on a rimmed baking sheet and transfer it to the oven.

Bake, rotating once, until the quiches are puffy and brown and a toothpick inserted into the center comes out clean, 18 to 20 minutes. Serve warm.

Store leftovers in an airtight container in the refrigerator for up to 3 days. Simply reheat in the oven at 325°F until warmed through, about 10 minutes.

Nutritional analysis per serving (1 mini quiche): *Calories 145, Fat 9 g, Saturated Fat 2 g, Cholesterol 300 mg, Fiber 2 g, Protein 11 g, Carbohydrates 8 g, Sodium 586 mg*

ROASTED VEGETABLES WITH ARTICHOKE HUMMUS

Serves: 8

Prep Time:
15 minutes

Cook Time:
30 minutes

Artichokes are one of my favorite vegetables because they peak during the winter, yet there is something very light and springlike about them. This twist on hummus substitutes artichokes for chickpeas to yield that creaminess we all love. Along with great flavor and texture, this recipe boasts healthy amounts of fiber and is sure to satisfy you for hours until your next meal.

- 1 large head cauliflower, cored and cut into 2-inch florets
- ½ cup plus 2 tablespoons extra-virgin olive oil
- 1 pound asparagus, trimmed
- 8 ounces green beans, trimmed
- 10 ounces Brussels sprouts, trimmed and halved
- 10 ounces cherry tomatoes
- 2 (9-ounce) packages frozen artichoke hearts, thawed
- 2 garlic cloves, halved
- ¼ cup tahini
- grated zest and juice of 1 lemon
- 1 tablespoon chopped fresh parsley
- ½ teaspoon sea salt
- ¼ teaspoon freshly ground black pepper
- ¼ teaspoon ground cumin

Preheat the oven to 450°F. Line two rimmed baking sheets with foil.

In a large bowl, toss the cauliflower with 2 tablespoons of the oil. Transfer the cauliflower to one of the lined baking sheets and roast until tender, 15 to 20 minutes. Place half of the cauliflower in a food processor and the other half on a platter.

Toss the asparagus, green beans, Brussels sprouts, and tomatoes with ¼ cup of the olive oil and divide between the two lined baking sheets. Roast until the vegetables are crisp-tender and beginning to brown, 10 to 15 minutes. Transfer to the platter with the cauliflower and let cool.

Meanwhile, to the food processor add the artichoke hearts, garlic, tahini, lemon zest and juice, and the remaining ¼ cup of the olive oil.

Puree, scraping down the sides occasionally, until smooth. Add the parsley, salt, black pepper, and cumin and continue to puree until well combined.

Serve the roasted vegetables with the artichoke dip. Store any leftover dip in an airtight container in the refrigerator for up to 5 days.

Nutritional analysis per serving: *Calories: 290, Fat: 22 g, Saturated Fat: 3.5 g, Cholesterol: 0 mg, Fiber: 10 g, Protein: 7 g, Carbohydrates: 20 g, Sodium: 160 mg*

SARDINE-CUCUMBER BITES

Sardines are a good source of omega-3 fatty acids without the mercury levels seen in larger fish. Enjoy a bit of the olive oil they are packed in for extra healthy fat.

- 2 tablespoons fresh lemon juice
- 1 tablespoon Mayonnaise (page 299) or Vegenaise
- 2 tablespoons finely chopped fresh chives, plus more for garnish
- 1 tablespoon capers, rinsed, drained, and chopped
- 1 teaspoon smoked paprika, plus more for garnish
- 1 (6.7-ounce) can oil-packed wild sardines, flaked into small pieces, oil reserved
- 1 small red bell pepper, seeded and finely chopped
- 1 seedless cucumber, trimmed and sliced

Combine the lemon juice, mayonnaise, chives, capers, and paprika in a large bowl.

Fold in the sardines and bell pepper and gently mix. Add 1 tablespoon of oil from the sardine can if the mixture is dry.

Mound the sardine mixture onto the cucumber slices and garnish with additional paprika. Serve.

Nutritional analysis per serving: Calories: 140 Fat: 8 g, Saturated Fat: 1 g, Cholesterol: 70 mg, Fiber: 1 g, Protein: 13 g, Carbohydrates: 4 g, Sodium: 340 mg

CREAMY HERBED TAHINI DIP

Makes: about
2 cups

Prep Time:
15 minutes

Tahini is a key ingredient in hummus and falafel, and is also used to make many other sauces and dips. It's rich, creamy, and very nutritious. Serve this dip with raw vegetables (such as celery, cucumbers, grape tomatoes, broccoli, snow peas, broccolini, and haricots verts) or as a sauce over grilled fish.

- 1 cup tahini
- ¼ cup loosely packed fresh cilantro leaves
- 8 to 10 fresh mint leaves
- 5 large fresh basil leaves
- 1 large scallion, cut into 2-inch pieces
- 2 tablespoons minced fresh chives
- 1 garlic clove, halved
- juice of 1 lemon
- 2 tablespoons extra-virgin olive oil
- ½ teaspoon sea salt
- ¼ teaspoon ground turmeric
- ¼ teaspoon ground cumin
- ¼ teaspoon ground coriander
- ¼ teaspoon fennel or anise seeds

Combine all of the ingredients plus 1 cup of hot water in a blender and blend until smooth. Add more hot water as needed if the blender is struggling. Serve.

Store any leftover dip in an airtight container in the refrigerator for up to 5 days.

Nutritional analysis per serving (2 tablespoons): *Calories: 105, Fat: 10 g, Saturated Fat: 1 g, Cholesterol: 0 mg, Fiber: 1 g, Protein: 3 g, Carbohydrates: 4 g, Sodium: 79 mg*

SPICY ROASTED PEPPER AND WALNUT DIP

Makes: about
2 cups

Prep Time:
10 minutes

Cook Time:
30 minutes

Here's a great snack to serve with carrots, radishes, sugar snap peas, celery, jicama, or any other favorite crunchy fresh vegetable.

- 2 tablespoons extra-virgin olive oil
- 4 red bell peppers, seeded and cut into ½-inch-thick strips
- ¼ cup shelled walnuts
- ½ to ¾ teaspoon crushed red pepper flakes
- ¼ teaspoon sea salt

Preheat the oven to 500°F.

Line two rimmed baking sheets with aluminum foil and brush with the oil. Spread the bell peppers out on the sheets and roast until they are tender and browning at the edges, 17 to 20 minutes.

Transfer the peppers to a food processor and process until smooth. Add the walnuts, crushed red pepper flakes, and salt and process again until smooth. Serve.

Store any leftover dip in an airtight container in the refrigerator for up to 5 days.

Nutritional analysis per serving (¼ cup): *Calories: 70, Fat: 6 g, Saturated Fat: 0.5 g, Cholesterol: 0 mg, Fiber: 1 g, Protein: 1 g, Carbohydrates: 4 g, Sodium: 75 mg*

BABA GHANOUSH

Baba ghanoush is a traditional Middle Eastern eggplant dip that is rich in vitamins, minerals, and important phytonutrients.

- 2 small eggplants
- ¼ cup tahini
- 2 tablespoons extra-virgin olive oil
- 2 garlic cloves, halved
- juice of 1 lemon
- ½ teaspoon sea salt
- ¼ cup loosely packed coarsely chopped parsley
- 1 bunch celery, cut into sticks, for serving

Serves: 8

Prep Time: 10 minutes, plus cooling time

Cook Time: 55 minutes

Preheat the broiler. Line a rimmed baking sheet with foil.

Prick each eggplant a few times with a fork and place on the lined baking sheet. Place the eggplants about 4 inches under the broiler and broil, turning every 5 minutes or so, until the skin is completely charred, 15 to 20 minutes. Remove from the oven and heat the oven to 375°F.

When the oven comes to temperature, return the eggplants to the oven and roast until they are completely soft, 30 to 35 minutes; when pressed with the back of a fork they should offer little resistance.

Allow the eggplants to cool enough so that you can handle them, about 25 minutes.

Cut each eggplant in half and, using a rubber spatula, carefully scrape out the pulp. Discard the skin.

In a blender or food processor, combine the eggplant pulp, tahini, olive oil, garlic, lemon juice, and salt. Puree until smooth. Transfer the dip to a serving bowl and stir in the parsley. Serve with celery sticks for dipping.

Store any leftover baba ghanoush in an airtight container in the refrigerator for up to 5 days.

Nutritional analysis per serving (¼ cup): *Calories: 120, Fat: 8 g, Saturated Fat: 1 g, Cholesterol: 0 mg, Fiber: 5 g, Protein: 3 g, Carbohydrates: 12 g, Sodium: 240 mg*

WARM HERBED OLIVES

Serves: 8

Prep Time:
10 minutes

Try to find olives that have not been pitted, as they generally taste better and are of higher quality than pitted olives.

- ½ cup extra-virgin olive oil
- 2 garlic cloves, lightly crushed
- 1 (2-inch) strip lemon peel
- 1 bay leaf
- 6 to 8 black peppercorns
- ½ teaspoon dried rosemary or thyme
- ½ teaspoon fennel seeds
- 2 cups mixed unpitted olives

In a small saucepan, combine all of the ingredients except the olives. Over very low heat, warm the oil just until the garlic starts to gently sizzle, then remove from the heat.

Place the olives in a glass or ceramic bowl and pour the warm oil over them. Allow the olives to marinate at room temperature for 1 hour before serving.

Store any leftover olives in an airtight container in the refrigerator for up to 2 weeks; allow to come to room temperature before serving.

Nutritional analysis per serving (¼ cup): *Calories: 159, Fat: 16 g, Saturated Fat: 2 g, Cholesterol: 0 mg, Fiber: 1 g, Protein: 1 g, Carbohydrates: 4 g, Sodium: 517 mg*

GUA-KALE-MOLE

Serves: 6

Prep Time:
15 minutes

If you have picky eaters around, this recipe is one you will want to whip up soon! They won't even know they are eating healthy greens with each delicious, delectable bite. Serve with fresh veggie dippers such as cucumbers, radishes, sugar snap peas, cherry tomatoes, cauliflowers, red bell peppers, and carrots.

- 2 bunches kale, stemmed and roughly chopped
- 1 bunch cilantro, stems included
- 2 tomatoes, chopped
- ⅓ red onion, chopped
- 1 jalapeño, seeded and halved
- 1 garlic clove, halved
- juice of 2 limes
- ½ teaspoon sea salt
- 3 avocados, peeled and pitted

In the bowl of a food processor, combine the kale, cilantro, 1 cup of the chopped tomato, 1½ tablespoons of the onion, the jalapeño, garlic, lime juice, and salt. Puree the mixture until smooth, scraping down the sides as needed, 1 to 2 minutes. Add the avocados and puree again until blended, 30 seconds to 1 minute.

Transfer the gua-kale-mole to a bowl and stir in the remaining chopped tomatoes and onion. Serve.

Store any leftover dip in an airtight container, with parchment paper pressed against the surface to prevent discoloration, in the refrigerator for up to 5 days.

Nutritional analysis per serving (½ cup): *Calories: 216, Fat: 15 g, Saturated Fat: 2 g, Cholesterol: 0 mg, Fiber: 10 g, Protein: 6 g, Carbohydrates: 20 g, Sodium: 235 mg*

CINNAMON AND CAYENNE ROASTED MIXED NUTS

Serves: 18

Prep Time:
10 minutes

Cook Time:
30 minutes

Try this sweet and spicy version of roasted nuts in place of your normal mid-morning snack.

- 1½ cups raw pecan halves
- 1½ cups raw cashews
- 1½ cups raw almonds
- 3 tablespoons coconut oil
- 1½ teaspoons ground cinnamon
- 1 teaspoon ground sweet paprika
- ½ to 1 teaspoon cayenne pepper
- ½ teaspoon sea salt
- ¼ teaspoon freshly ground black pepper

Preheat the oven to 350°F. Line a baking sheet with aluminum foil.

In a large bowl, combine the pecans, cashews, and almonds. In a small bowl, combine the coconut oil, cinnamon, paprika, cayenne, salt, and black pepper.

Pour the spiced coconut oil over the nuts in the large bowl. Using your hands or a large spoon, toss the nuts in the spiced oil, making sure to evenly coat all of the nuts. Spread the nuts in an even layer on the lined baking sheet.

Bake the nuts, stirring and tossing occasionally, until toasted, 25 to 30 minutes.

Remove the nuts from the oven and let them cool to room temperature. Serve.

Store any leftover nuts in an airtight container in the refrigerator for up to 5 days.

Nutritional analysis per serving (¼ cup nuts): *Calories: 206, Fat: 19 g, Saturated Fat: 4 g, Cholesterol: 0 mg, Fiber: 3 g, Protein: 5 g, Carbohydrates: 8 g, Sodium: 66 mg*

ROASTED GARLIC WITH OLIVE OIL AND ROSEMARY

When a whole head of garlic is roasted slowly in the oven, the garlic softens and sweetens into a mild, creamy paste. It loses all its sharp pungency, and mellows out into a fragrant, gentler version of itself. Roasted garlic can be used as a spread, mixed into sauces and dressings, or added to pureed vegetables and soups.

- 2 heads garlic, unpeeled
- 2 teaspoons extra-virgin olive oil
- 1 rosemary sprig

Preheat the oven to 400°F.

Using a serrated knife, slice both heads of garlic crosswise so you have top and bottom layers, even in size.

Rub each of the four cut surfaces with the olive oil, and then place the garlic and rosemary on a sheet of aluminum foil. Wrap the garlic and rosemary in the foil to seal it up tightly, then place it directly on a rack in the oven.

Roast the garlic until it is very soft and fragrant, about 45 minutes; when you peek inside the foil, you should see that the cut edges are turning golden brown.

Allow the heads to cool enough to handle, then squeeze the roasted garlic from the cloves and use as needed.

Store any leftover roasted garlic in an airtight container in the refrigerator for up to 5 days.

Nutritional analysis per serving (1 tablespoon): *Calories: 29, Fat: 2 g, Saturated Fat: 0 g, Cholesterol: 0 mg, Fiber: 0 g, Protein: 1 g, Carbohydrates: 3 g, Sodium: 2 mg*

Makes: about ⅓ cup

Prep Time: 5 minutes

Cook Time: 45 minutes

LEMONY CASHEW-TAHINI DIP

Serves: 4

Prep Time:
10 minutes,
plus soaking
time

This thick, hummus-style dip tastes great with raw veggie dippers, such as broccoli, carrots, red bell peppers, or sugar snap peas. If you add even more water, you can thin the dip into a dressing, which pairs well with kale and other hearty greens.

- 1 cup raw cashews
- ¼ cup tahini
- juice of 1 lemon
- ¼ teaspoon sea salt

Put the cashews in a bowl and cover with at least 1 cup of warm water. Let sit until softened, 20 to 30 minutes.

Use a slotted spoon to transfer the soaked cashews to a food processor, making sure to reserve the cashew soaking water. Add the tahini, lemon juice, and salt to the food processor and puree the mixture, adding ¼ cup of the reserved cashew water through the feed tube as it is processing. If necessary, add another few tablespoons of the water until the dip is the consistency of hummus. (For a thinner dressing, add up to ½ cup more of the reserved water, a few tablespoons at a time, until the desired consistency is achieved.) Serve.

Store any leftover dip or dressing in an airtight container in the refrigerator for 3 to 5 days.

Nutritional analysis per serving (¼ cup): *Calories: 270, Fat: 22 g, Saturated Fat: 4 g, Cholesterol: 0 mg, Fiber: 2 g, Protein: 9 g, Carbohydrates: 14 g, Sodium: 156 mg*

SAUCES AND CONDIMENTS

MIXED BERRY SALSA

Serves: 4

Prep Time: 15 minutes

Sneaking low-glycemic berries into what are normally vegetable-based recipes provides a touch of sweetness without the harm of refined sugar. Serve this salsa with fresh vegetables such as cucumber slices, cauliflower florets, and radishes.

- 1 cup chopped strawberries
- ½ cup blueberries
- ½ cup raspberries
- 1 medium tomato, cored and chopped
- ⅓ red onion, chopped
- 1 or 2 jalapeños, seeded and finely chopped
- ½ bunch cilantro, stemmed and chopped
- 2 tablespoons fresh lime juice
- ¼ teaspoon sea salt

Combine all of the ingredients in a medium bowl, stirring gently to combine. Serve. Store any leftover salsa in an airtight container in the refrigerator for up to 5 days.

Nutritional analysis per serving (½ cup): *Calories: 45, Fat: 0 g, Saturated Fat: 0 g, Cholesterol: 0 mg, Fiber: 3 g, Protein: 1 g, Carbohydrates: 11 g, Sodium: 150 mg*

MARINARA SAUCE

Serves: 4

Prep Time:
10 minutes

Cook Time:
40 minutes

This basic tomato sauce can be served over steamed vegetables or blanched shirataki noodles for a quick lunch or dinner option.

- 1½ teaspoons olive oil
- 1 medium yellow onion, finely chopped
- 2 garlic cloves, minced
- 1 (28-ounce) can diced tomatoes
- 2 bay leaves
- ¾ teaspoon dried oregano
- ½ teaspoon dried thyme
- ½ teaspoon dried basil
- ½ teaspoon sea salt
- ¼ teaspoon freshly ground black pepper
- 2 tablespoons chopped fresh basil

In a heavy pot, heat the oil over medium-high heat until shimmering. Add the onion and cook, stirring frequently, until softened, 8 to 10 minutes.

Add the garlic and cook, stirring, for 30 seconds. Add the tomatoes with their juices, bay leaves, dried herbs, salt, and black pepper. Stir to combine. Let the sauce come to a boil and then reduce the heat to a simmer. Partially cover the pot and cook the sauce 30 minutes.

Remove the bay leaves and serve, garnished with the fresh basil. Store any leftover sauce in an airtight container in the refrigerator for up to 5 days.

Nutritional analysis per serving (¾ cup): Calories: 73, Fat: 2 g, Saturated Fat: 0 g, Cholesterol: 0 mg, Fiber: 2 g, Protein: 2 g, Carbohydrates: 12 g, Sodium: 313 mg

SESAME-COCONUT CURRY SAUCE

Serves: 8

Prep Time:
15 minutes

Cook Time:
15 minutes

This peanut-free version of a classic Asian sauce can be served with grilled chicken sate, steamed vegetables, or spring rolls. Almond butter replaces the peanut butter, but you could substitute cashew butter or sunflower butter, too. The sauce keeps well in the refrigerator for up to 5 days; reheat it gently over low heat, mixing in a little warm water to loosen the sauce if necessary.

- 1 tablespoon grapeseed oil
- 1 large garlic clove, minced
- 1 (2-inch) piece ginger, peeled and grated
- 2 teaspoons curry powder
- ½ teaspoon ground turmeric
- ¼ teaspoon cayenne pepper (optional)
- 1 (13.5-ounce) can full-fat unsweetened coconut milk
- ¼ cup tahini
- ¼ cup almond butter
- 1 tablespoon gluten-free, low-sodium tamari
- ½ teaspoon toasted sesame oil
- 1 tablespoon fresh lime juice

Warm the grapeseed oil in a saucepan over low heat. Add the garlic and ginger and sauté until soft and very fragrant, about 3 minutes. Add the curry powder, turmeric, and cayenne (if using) and sauté for another minute to toast the spices.

Add the coconut milk and whisk the sauce well to combine. Raise the heat to medium and simmer until the coconut milk has reduced in volume by one-third, about 10 minutes.

Remove the pan from the heat and allow the sauce to cool for 5 minutes, then whisk in the tahini, almond butter, tamari, and sesame oil. Add the lime juice just before serving.

Store any leftover sauce in an airtight container in the refrigerator for up to 5 days.

Nutritional analysis per serving (¼ cup): *Calories: 210, Fat: 21 g, Saturated Fat: 10 g, Cholesterol: 0 mg, Fiber: 1 g, Protein: 4 g, Carbohydrates: 5 g, Sodium: 115 mg*

GREMOLATA WITH ALMONDS

Serves: 6

Prep Time:
5 minutes, plus
soaking time

Serve this refreshing condiment over roasted carrots or roasted asparagus; it also works beautifully as a side dish to any entrée.

- 1 cup raw almonds
- 1 or 2 garlic cloves, halved
- 2 bunches parsley, stemmed
- grated zest of 2 lemons
- 1 teaspoon fresh lemon juice
- ¼ teaspoon sea salt
- pinch of freshly ground black pepper

Soak the almonds in a small bowl of warm water until softened, about 30 minutes.

Drain the almonds and transfer to a food processor. Process until finely ground, about 1 minute. Add the garlic, parsley, lemon zest, lemon juice, salt, and black pepper and process until the mixture is crumbly and finely chopped, 30 seconds to 1 minute. Serve.

Store any leftover gremolata in an airtight container in the refrigerator for up to 5 days.

Nutritional analysis per serving (¼ cup): Calories: 150, Fat: 12 g, Saturated Fat: 1 g, Cholesterol: 0 mg, Fiber: 4 g, Protein: 6 g, Carbohydrates: 7 g, Sodium: 110 mg

KALE PESTO

Baby kale makes for a fun alternative to traditional basil pesto. The lemon zest and juice bring a fresh, bright flavor to the pesto while keeping it dairy-free.

- 1 garlic clove, halved
- 2 tablespoons pine nuts
- grated zest and juice of 1 large lemon
- 5 ounces baby kale
- ¼ cup extra-virgin olive oil
- ¼ teaspoon sea salt
- ¼ teaspoon freshly ground black pepper

In a food processor, pulse the garlic and pine nuts until finely chopped. Add the lemon zest and juice. Add the kale and pulse until coarsely chopped. With the machine running, add the oil through the feed tube and puree until almost smooth. Season with the salt and black pepper and puree again.

Store any leftover pesto in an airtight container in the refrigerator for up to 5 days.

Nutritional analysis per serving (¼ cup): *Calories: 110, Fat: 11 g, Saturated Fat: 1.5 g, Cholesterol: 0 mg, Fiber: 1 g, Protein: 1 g, Carbohydrates: 2 g, Sodium: 100 mg*

CHIMICHURRI

Serves: 6

Prep Time:
10 minutes

This green sauce originated in Argentina and is traditionally served on meat. This version, packed with citrus and fresh herb flavors, works well on fish and chicken, too.

- 2 bunches parsley, stemmed
- 1 bunch cilantro, stems included
- ½ bunch mint, stemmed
- 2 oil-packed anchovies
- 1 tablespoon capers, rinsed
- 1 garlic clove, halved
- 2 tablespoons extra-virgin olive oil
- grated zest and juice of ½ lemon
- ¼ teaspoon sea salt
- pinch of freshly ground black pepper

Combine all of the ingredients in a food processor and blend until smooth. Store any leftover sauce in an airtight container in the refrigerator for up to 5 days.

Nutritional analysis per serving (2 tablespoons): *Calories: 50, Fat: 5 g, Saturated Fat: 0.5 g, Cholesterol: 0 mg, Fiber: 1 g, Protein: 1 g, Carbohydrates: 2 g, Sodium: 200 mg*

CASHEW "RICOTTA CHEESE"

Makes: about
2 cups

Prep Time:
5 minutes, plus
soaking time

Cashews contain magnesium, copper, manganese, zinc, healthy essential fatty acids, and protein, and they tend to be hypoallergenic so most people can tolerate them easily. Serve this spread with fresh vegetables such as bell peppers, celery, or snap peas as a healthy alternative to dairy cheese.

- 2 cups raw cashews
- 2 tablespoon extra-virgin olive oil
- 4 teaspoons fresh lemon juice
- 1 teaspoon sea salt

Soak the cashews in a bowl of hot water for at least 1 hour at room temperature or up to 24 hours in the refrigerator. Drain the cashews and place them in a food processor, along with the olive oil, lemon juice, salt, and ¼ cup of warm water. Process the ingredients until a smooth paste forms; you may need to add a bit more water, depending on how long you soaked the cashews. Serve.

Store any leftover "cheese" in an airtight container in the refrigerator for up to 3 days.

Nutritional analysis per serving (¼ cup): *Calories: 210, Fat: 18 g, Saturated Fat: 3 g, Cholesterol: 0 mg, Fiber: 1 g, Protein: 6 g, Carbohydrates: 11 g, Sodium: 290 mg*

SPICY TOMATILLO-AVOCADO SAUCE

Serves: 6

Prep Time:
10 minutes

Cook Time:
15 minutes

This sauce, when chilled, is a wonderful substitute for sour cream in Tex-Mex dishes, and it adds a bit of richness as a garnish for a pureed vegetable soup. It also takes well to the addition of spices, so feel free to change it up a bit. I like to add cumin, chili powder, or curry powder. Try experimenting with your favorite spices.

- 4 small tomatillos, husks removed
- 1 jalapeño, seeded and halved
- 1 avocado, peeled and pitted
- juice of 1 lime
- ¼ teaspoon sea salt

Fill a 3-quart saucepan with water and add the tomatillos and jalapeño. Bring the water to a boil over medium-high heat, then reduce to a simmer and cook until the tomatillos are tender, 7 to 10 minutes. With a slotted spoon, transfer the tomatillos and jalapeño to a blender, and puree until smooth. Add the avocado, lime juice, and salt and continue to puree until a thick sauce forms. Serve.

Store any leftover sauce in an airtight container, with parchment paper pressed against the surface of the sauce to prevent discoloration, for up to 3 days.

Nutritional analysis per serving (¼ cup): *Calories: 60, Fat: 5 g, Saturated Fat: 0.5 g, Cholesterol: 0 mg, Fiber: 3 g, Protein: 1 g, Carbohydrates: 5 g, Sodium: 105 mg*

Salsa Roja

Serve this salsa as a dip with cucumber slices and other mild vegetables. It is also great swirled into soup, used as a salad dressing, or spooned over meat.

- 6 dried chiles (such as guajillo, California, pasilla, and/or New Mexican)
- 3 tomatoes, roughly chopped
- 2 tablespoons chopped red onion
- 1 garlic clove, halved
- 1½ tablespoons cider vinegar
- ¼ teaspoon sea salt

Put the dried chiles in a bowl and add enough boiling water to cover. Soak them until softened, 20 to 30 minutes.

Remove the chiles from the bowl with a slotted spoon, reserving ¼ cup of the soaking water.

Peel open the chiles and remove the stems and seeds. Put the chiles in a food processor, along with the tomatoes, onion, garlic, vinegar, and salt. Process the mixture, adding the reserved ¼ cup chile soaking water through the feed tube. Blend until the salsa is smooth, 1 to 2 minutes. Serve.

Store any leftover salsa in an airtight container in the refrigerator for up to 5 days.

Nutritional analysis per serving (½ cup): *Calories: 35, Fat: 0 g, Saturated Fat: 0 g, Cholesterol: 0 mg, Fiber: 1 g, Protein: 1 g, Carbohydrates: 7 g, Sodium: 160 mg*

ROASTED PEPPER AND RED ONION RELISH

Makes: about
2 cups

Prep Time:
20 minutes

Cook Time:
12 hours
(unattended),
plus 30 minutes

Impress your guests the next time you have company over with this savory, slightly sweet relish. Spread it on top of fresh vegetables or use it to dress up a plain roast chicken or steamed fish. If you don't have a slow cooker, you can bake the roasted vegetables in a covered Dutch oven at 300°F for 3½ hours.

- 6 red bell peppers, seeded and cut into ½-inch-thick strips
- 2 jalapeños, seeded and thinly sliced (optional)
- 5 red onions, cut crosswise into ½-inch-thick slices and separated into rings
- 4 tablespoons extra-virgin olive oil
- sea salt

Preheat the oven to 500°F.

Line two rimmed baking sheets with aluminum foil. Place half of the peppers and onions on the baking sheets and toss the vegetables on each sheet with 1 tablespoon of the olive oil and a pinch of salt. Roast the peppers and onions until they are tender and browning at the edges, 15 to 17 minutes, rotating the sheets halfway through cooking. Transfer the vegetables to a 6-quart slow cooker.

Roast the second batch of peppers and onions in the same way, again tossing each sheet with 1 tablespoon of the olive oil and a pinch of salt. Transfer to the slow cooker.

Once all of the vegetables have been added, cook on low for 12 hours. Serve.

Store any leftover relish in an airtight container in the refrigerator for up to 2 weeks.

Nutritional analysis per serving (¼ cup): *Calories: 150, Fat: 10 g, Saturated Fat: 1.5 g, Cholesterol: 0 mg, Fiber: 4 g, Protein: 2 g, Carbohydrates: 16 g, Sodium: 200 mg*

MAYONNAISE

Makes: about
1 cup

Prep Time:
5 minutes

Homemade mayo tastes so much better than the kind from a jar, and if you make it in the blender, it's super fast! Since raw eggs are used, be sure to buy organic eggs for this recipe.

- 1 large omega-3 egg
- 4 teaspoons fresh lemon juice
- 1 teaspoon Dijon mustard
- ¼ teaspoon sea salt
- ¼ teaspoon freshly ground black pepper
- 1 cup extra-virgin olive oil

In a blender or food processor, combine the egg, lemon juice, mustard, salt, and black pepper and blend until well combined, 1 to 2 minutes.

With the blender still running, slowly add the oil in a steady stream through the hole in the lid and continue to blend until the mayo is thick and smooth. Serve.

Store any leftover mayonnaise in an airtight container in the refrigerator for up to 1 week.

Nutritional analysis per serving (1 tablespoon): *Calories: 125, Fat: 14 g, Saturated Fat: 2 g, Cholesterol: 14 mg, Fiber: 0 g, Protein: 1 g, Carbohydrates: 0 g, Sodium: 45 mg*

SPICES, RUBS, AND STOCKS

Ras el Hanout

Makes: about
3 tablespoons

Prep Time:
5 minutes

Ras el hanout is a Middle Eastern spice mix available at specialty markets, but it's easy enough to make your own. Use this in the Pomegranate Chicken recipe (page 188); it also makes a tasty rub for all kinds of meat, poultry, and fish.

- 2 teaspoons ground cumin
- 1 teaspoon ground ginger
- 1 teaspoon ground cinnamon
- 1 teaspoon ground coriander
- 1 teaspoon sea salt
- ¾ teaspoon freshly ground black pepper
- ½ teaspoon cayenne pepper
- ½ teaspoon ground allspice

Combine all of the ingredients in a small bowl and mix well. Store in an airtight container in a cool, dark place for up to 1 month.

Nutritional analysis per serving (1 teaspoon): Calories: 5, Fat: 0 g, Saturated Fat: 0 g, Cholesterol: 0 mg, Fiber: 1 g, Protein: 0 g, Carbohydrates: 1 g, Sodium: 290 mg

DR. HYMAN'S GO-TO SPICE RUB

Makes: about ¼ cup

Prep Time: 5 minutes

Keep a batch of this spice rub easily accessible in your pantry to elevate any weeknight meal featuring fish, poultry, or meat to an extraordinary dining experience.

- 2 teaspoons ground turmeric
- 2 teaspoons smoked or sweet paprika
- 2 teaspoons ground coriander
- 2 teaspoons ground cumin
- 2 teaspoons ground ginger
- ½ teaspoon ground cloves
- 2 teaspoons sea salt

Combine all of the ingredients in a small bowl and mix well. Store in an airtight container in a cool, dark place for up to 1 month.

Nutritional analysis per serving (1 teaspoon): *Calories: 5, fat: 0 g, Saturated Fat: 0 g, Cholesterol: 0 mg, Fiber: 0 g, Protein: 0 g, Carbohydrates: 1 g, Sodium: 382 mg*

THAI GREEN CURRY PASTE

Makes: about
¾ cup

Prep Time:
20 minutes

Cook Time:
3 minutes

Full of spice and flavor, this paste is perfect in my Thai Green Curry with Soft-Shell Crabs (page 143).

- 1 tablespoon coriander seeds
- 1 tablespoon cumin seeds
- ½ teaspoon black peppercorns
- 4 to 6 green Thai or serrano chiles, seeded
- 1 lemongrass stalk, roughly chopped
- 3 large shallots, roughly chopped
- 15 garlic cloves, halved
- 3 (2-inch) pieces ginger, peeled and roughly chopped
- 1 bunch parsley, stemmed
- 2 tablespoons fish sauce
- 1 teaspoon sea salt

Toast the coriander seeds, cumin seeds, and peppercorns in a large skillet over medium heat until fragrant and beginning to brown, 2 to 3 minutes, stirring constantly. Transfer to a plate to cool.

In a spice grinder, grind the cooled spices until a powder forms. Set aside.

In the bowl of a food processor, combine the chiles, lemongrass, shallots, garlic, ginger, parsley, fish sauce, and salt. Process, scraping down the sides of the bowl, until the mixture is a smooth paste, about 2 minutes. If the food processor begins to warm up (feel the side of the machine), give it a 5-minute break to cool down; do not overwork the engine. Once the mixture is smooth, add the ground spices and continue to process until combined.

Store the paste in an airtight container in the refrigerator for up to 7 days.

Nutritional analysis per serving (1 tablespoon): *Calories: 35, Fat: 0 g, Saturated Fat: 0 g, Cholesterol: 0 mg, Fiber: 1 g, Protein: 2 g, Carbohydrates: 7 g, Sodium: 582 mg*

HERB SALT

Makes: about
2 cups

Prep Time:
10 minutes

Cook Time:
2½ hours

Herb salt is a great way to customize your favorite dishes. You can use a variety of fresh herbs (experiment by mixing and matching) to make different blends that will add kick to vegetables, meat, and fish. The salt is quick to assemble and lasts a long time.

- 2 cups sea salt
- 3 tablespoons minced fresh thyme
- 1 tablespoon minced fresh rosemary
- 1 tablespoon minced fresh tarragon

Preheat the oven to 200°F.

Combine all of the ingredients in a bowl. Evenly spread the salt mixture on a rimmed baking sheet. Bake, stirring occasionally, until the herbs are no longer moist, about 2½ hours.

Allow the salt to cool completely, then transfer to an airtight container. Store in a cool, dark place for up 1 month.

Nutritional analysis per serving (¼ teaspoon): *Calories: 0, Fat: 0 g, Saturated Fat: 0 g, Cholesterol: 0 mg, Fiber: 0 g, Protein: 0 g, Carbohydrates: 0 g, Sodium: 480 mg.*

VEGETABLE-HERB STOCK

Serves: 4

Prep Time:
15 minutes

Cook Time:
1 hour and
15 minutes

Food is medicine, and the most flavorful ingredients add pleasure to our palate as well as nutrition to our bodies. Making homemade stock is a simple, fun way to enjoy nutrient-dense ingredients. Make a double batch and store half in the freezer—once you taste it, you won't miss the store-bought version for a second.

- 2 fennel bulbs with fronds, sliced
- 2 carrots, roughly chopped
- 2 yellow onions, roughly chopped
- 10 ounces cremini mushrooms, trimmed and halved
- 2 ounces spinach or other greens
- 5 garlic cloves, halved
- 1 bunch parsley, stems included
- 1 large rosemary sprig
- 5 to 6 thyme sprigs
- 2 bay leaves
- 1 teaspoon sea salt
- 1 teaspoon black peppercorns
- 1 teaspoon coconut aminos or gluten-free, low-sodium tamari

Combine all of the ingredients in a large stockpot. Add 10 to 12 cups of water to the pot, enough to cover the vegetables. Don't worry about some veggies poking out; they will sink down during the cooking.

Bring the water to a boil over high heat; reduce the heat to a simmer and cook for 60 to 75 minutes.

Let the stock cool a bit, then strain out the solids by pouring the stock through a colander placed over a large bowl or pot. Discard the solids.

Pour the vegetable stock into airtight containers and store in the refrigerator for up to 3 days or in the freezer for up to 6 months.

Nutritional analysis per serving (1 cup): *Calories: 5, Fat: 0 g, Saturated Fat: 0 g, Cholesterol: 0 mg, Fiber: 0 g, Protein: 0 g, Carbohydrates: 2 g, Sodium: 200 mg*

8

Healthy Meal Plans

Now that you have the tools and tips and have been introduced to all these new ingredients, you might be wondering which meals work best together to create complete meals. I hope the following suggestions help you create delicious meal plans for your family and friends. *Bon appétit!*

LUNCH AND DINNER IDEAS

Creamy Herbed Tahini Dip, Arugula and Fennel Salad, and Ginger-Lemon Chicken with Spinach

Heirloom Tomato, Cucumber, and Radish Salad, steamed carrots with Gremolata with Almonds, and Lebanese-Style Lamb Stew

Onion-Leek Soup, Niçoise Salad with Poached Salmon, and Bell Pepper Mini Quiches

Chicken Spring Rolls with Almond Sauce, Spicy Garlic Eggplant with Mint, and Thai Green Curry with Soft-Shell Crabs

Taco Salad with Flank Steak, Spicy Cauliflower Sauté, and Spicy Mocktail

Thai Tofu and Avocado Salad with Chile-Lime Dressing, Fried "Rice" with Shrimp, and Asian-Spiced Salmon Cakes

Deviled Eggs, Moroccan Chicken and Vegetable Stew, and Steamed Vegetables with Lemon Aioli

Roasted Vegetables with Artichoke Hummus, Zucchini Ribbons with Pearl Onions and Cardamom, Miso-Marinated Cod with Fresh Basil and Bok Choy, and Cauliflower "Rice"

Warm Herbed Olives, Stuffed Campari Tomatoes, and Chili-Spiced Turkey Meatloaf with Roasted Carrot Salad

BRUNCH IDEAS

Blueberry-Nut Smoothie, Cherry Tomato and Tofu Salad, and Vegetable Hash with Fried Eggs

Açai Smoothie, Crustless Asparagus Quiche, and Turkey Sausage Patties

Jicama Fries, Chicken Salad in Endive Cups, Spinach-Mushroom-Asparagus Strata, and Creamy Berry Smoothie

Heirloom Tomato, Cucumber, and Radish Salad, Garlic and Chile Broccolini with Soft-Boiled Eggs, and Almond-Berry Smoothie

Egg Salad in Endive Spears, Grilled Chicken with Basil Pesto, and Strawberry-Almond-Coconut Smoothie

AFTER THE 10-DAY DETOX DIET

Congratulations! You have given yourself a gift—the gift of real food and optimal health. The main idea behind *The 10-Day Detox Diet* and *The 10-Day Detox Diet Cookbook* is to help you connect the dots between what you eat and how you feel, and to provide a way for you to experience the power of food as medicine. But now what? Now you can reintroduce foods (but only real foods) to your diet and monitor how you feel. I hope you never go back to eating processed, industrial science projects masquerading as food, or to pharmacological doses of sugar and flour. My hope is that you stick with real, whole, fresh food. My hope is for you to introduce beans, grains, and even small amounts of dairy and gluten and sugar (as a treat) and see how you feel. You now have a fresh start, an opportunity to transition to a new way of eating and to notice how your body likes (or doesn't) certain foods, like gluten and dairy.

Depending on your goals, there are different options for transitioning off *The 10-Day Detox Diet*. I have created a free downloadable guide—*The 10-Day Detox Diet Cookbook Companion Guide*—with detailed guidelines on how to transition safely while enjoying a wide variety of delicious foods. The guide includes instructions on how to discover which transition plan is best for you, how to safely reintroduce foods without getting sick, and how to track their effects on your health. And I have also included a few delicious, easy recipes for the Transition Phase. Please go to www.10daydetox.com/tools to download your free guide!

This book is meant to help you figure out how to change your life through food. Whether you are just beginning to experiment with simple ways to prepare basic foods or expanding your repertoire to include new tastes and ingredients, I hope this book provides the road map, the tools and the inspiration. I had two main goals in writing this book.

First, I want to encourage you to cook real, delicious, and inspiring meals—for yourself, your family, or your entire community. As you stick to real foods prepared simply, you'll notice the pounds come off, the cravings disappear, and just about every aspect of your health improve.

And second, I want you to feel so great after the 10 days that you'll never want to return to the food desert from which you came. You will want to stay nourished and healthy. You'll want to continue healing yourself, your family, and your community through food. And not just for 10 days, but for the rest of your life.

After all, better health doesn't start and end in 10 days. It's a life-long journey. I've set out to make that journey both doable and delicious. Bon voyage, and *bon appétit!*

Acknowledgments

This cookbook is the work of many passionate souls who love food and are committed to transforming how we grow, produce, and consume food.

The vision started with one mission: to create simple, delicious, healing meals that help people experience the power of food. The power of food to delight the palate, invigorate the senses, and reboot the body. The power of real, whole, fresh food to help people see the connection between what they eat and how they feel, and realize that they are only ten days away from health and happiness.

But to do that, I needed to create inspired and delectable recipes that are easy and fun to make. So I gathered an amazing team. The team was led by Anne McLaughlin, who ensured that everything made sense and kept me on track. Lizzy Swick provided the oversight to make sure that my vision of healing, detoxifying ingredients was incorporated into each and every recipe. Lauren Zander and Amy Teuteberg created the Dinner Conversations, a way to bring love and connection and laughter into every meal.

Most important, the team at Luvo designed and created the healing recipes. Thank you, team Luvo: Christine Day, Chief Executive Officer; Stephen Sidwell, Founder; John Mitchell, Chief Innovation Officer and Executive Chef; Samantha Cassetty, Director of Nutrition; Margaret Wetzler, Director of Culinary Marketing; Eunice Choi, Project Manager, Culinary Marketing; Diane Maynard, Art Director; Diane Elander, Food Stylist; Bruce James, Photographer; Andrea Lynn, Emma Feigenbaum,

Erica Wides, and Genevieve Ko, Recipe Developers; and Brooks Halliday and Faryl Amadeus, Recipe Testers.

Of course, I could not have created all this without the love and support of my team at Little, Brown, especially my editor, Tracy Behar. Thank you for believing in the future of food and health and helping me make it a reality. My success is in large part because of my long-time believer, supporter, advocate, and agent, Richard Pine. Thank you for being part of the change.

Finally, thank *you* for taking back your kitchens, for taking a step closer to a vibrant, healthy life through the power of food. Cooking is the ultimate revolutionary act—food that we make ourselves can be simple, quick, inexpensive, and delicious. And cooking real food can transform everything that is ailing us as a society, because it changes how we produce and consume food—taking it out of the hands of Big Food and Big Ag and putting it back in your hands, where it belongs.

Resources

FURTHER READING AND RESOURCES FROM MARK HYMAN, MD

Mark Hyman's Websites
www.drhyman.com
www.10daydetox.com
www.bloodsugarsolution.com

The UltraWellness Center
55 Pittsfield Road, Suite 9
Lenox Commons
Lenox, MA 01240
(413) 637-9991
www.ultrawellnesscenter.com

I founded and am the medical director of this center. Our team of experienced functional medicine physicians, nutritionists, nurses, and health coaches guide you through diet and lifestyle modifications, as well as specialized testing, nutritional supplementation, and medications.

Cleveland Clinic Center for Functional Medicine
9500 Euclid Avenue / H-18
Cleveland, OH 44195
(216) 445-6900 or toll-free at (844) 833-0126

I am the director of this center. Our team of experienced functional medicine physicians, nutritionists, nurses, and health coaches guide you through diet and lifestyle modifications, as well as specialized testing, nutritional supplementation, and medications.

Books and Programs

The Blood Sugar Solution 10-Day Detox Diet (Book and Public Television Special)

www.10daydetox.com

The Blood Sugar Solution (Book and Public Television Special)

www.bloodsugarsolution.com

The UltraMind Solution (Book and Public Television Special)

Six Weeks to an UltraMind (Audio/DVD Program)

The Daniel Plan

www.danielplan.com

The Daniel Plan Cookbook

UltraCalm (Audio Program)

UltraMetabolism (Book and Public Television Special)

The UltraMetabolism Cookbook (Book)

The UltraSimple Diet (Book)

The UltraSimple Challenge (DVD Coaching Program)

The UltraThyroid Solution (Ebook)

UltraPrevention (Book)

Five Forces of Wellness (Audio Program)

The Detox Box (Audio/DVD Detoxification Program)

Nutrigenomics

GENERAL REFERENCES AND RESOURCES

Environmental Working Group

www.ewg.org

Environmental Working Group empowers people to live healthier lives in a healthier environment. They drive consumer choice and civic action with breakthrough research and an informed public. Use this site to download the guide "Good Food on a Tight Budget" and Clean Fifteen/Dirty Dozen produce lists. Download the Food Scores app to check your food for nutritional quality, ingredient check, and level of processing. You will also find guides for healthy fish, a guide to meat that is healthy for you and the planet, safe skin care and house-cleaning products, and more.

Organic Essentials

The Organic Pages

www.bloodsugarsolution.com/theorganicpages

The Organic Trade Association (OTA) provides users with a quick and easy way to find certified organic products, producers, ingredients, supplies, and services offered by OTA members, as well as items of interest to the entire organic community.

Organic Planet

organicplanet.com

Organic Planet is a leading supplier of natural and organic food ingredients.

Organic Provisions

www.bloodsugarsolution.com/orgfood

Organic Provisions is a convenient new way to choose a wide array of high-quality natural foods and products right from your home.

SunOrganic Farm

www.bloodsugarsolution.com/sunorganicfarm

SunOrganic Farm provides a direct source for online ordering of a wide variety of organic foods.

Produce

Earthbound Farm

www.ebfarm.com

Offers fresh, packaged organic produce.

Maine Coast Sea Vegetables

www.bloodsugarsolution.com/seaveg

A variety of sea vegetables, including some organically certified types.

Organic Frozen and Canned Foods

Cascadian Farm

www.bloodsugarsolution.com/cfarm

A great source of organic frozen fruit and vegetables.

Imagine Foods

www.bloodsugarsolution.com/imaginefoods

A high-quality purveyor of delicious organic soups.

Pacific Foods

www.bloodsugarsolution.com/pacificfoods

Pacific Foods carries high-quality soups, stocks, nut milk, hemp milk, and more.

Stahlbush Island Farms

www.bloodsugarsolution.com/stahlbush

An excellent source of sustainably grown frozen berries.

Meat, Poultry, and Eggs

Applegate Farms

www.bloodsugarsolution.com/applegatefarms

Natural and organic packaged poultry, meat, and deli products.

Eatwild

www.bloodsugarsolution.com/eatwild

Grass-fed meat.

Organic Valley

www.bloodsugarsolution.com/organicvalley

Organic meats, eggs, and produce from more than 600 member-owned organic farms.

Peaceful Pastures

www.bloodsugarsolution.com/peacefulpastures

Grass-fed and grass-finished meat and poultry products.

Pete and Gerry's Organic Eggs

www.bloodsugarsolution.com/peteandgerrys
Organic omega-3 eggs.

Fish

Crown Prince Natural

www.bloodsugarsolution.com/crownprince
Wild-caught, sustainably harvested canned seafood.

EcoFish

www.bloodsugarsolution.com/ecofish
Environmentally responsible seafood products and information.

SeaBear

www.bloodsugarsolution.com/seabear
Wild salmon jerky for a convenient snack.

Vital Choice

www.bloodsugarsolution.com/vitalchoice
A selection of fresh, frozen, and canned wild salmon, sardines, black cod, and small halibut.

Nuts, Seeds, and Oils

Barlean's Organic Oils

www.bloodsugarsolution.com/barleans
Organic oils and ground flaxseeds.

MaraNatha

www.bloodsugarsolution.com/maranthafoods
Organic nut and seed butters.

Omega Nutrition

www.bloodsugarsolution.com/omeganutrition
A variety of organic oils, flax, and hemp seed products.

Once Again

www.bloodsugarsolution.com/onceagainnutbutter
Organic nut and seed butters.

Spectrum Naturals

www.bloodsugarsolution.com/spectrumorganic
An extensive line of high-quality oils, vinegars, flaxseed products, and culinary resources.

Spices, Seasonings, Sauces, Soups, and Such

Edward & Sons

www.bloodsugarsolution.com/edwardandsons
An extensive line of vegetarian organic food products including miso, sauces, brown rice crackers, etc.

Flavorganics

www.bloodsugarsolution.com/flavorganics
A full product line of certified organic pure flavor extracts.

Frontier Co-Op

www.bloodsugarsolution.com/frontiernaturalbrands
An extensive line of organic spices, seasonings, baking flavors and extracts, dried foods, teas, and culinary gadgets.

Rapunzel

www.bloodsugarsolution.com/rapunzel
A great selection of seasonings.

Seeds of Change

www.bloodsugarsolution.com/seedsofchange
Organic tomato sauce, salsa, and more.

Spice Hunter

www.bloodsugarsolution.com/spicehunter
A complete line of organic spices.

Nondairy, Gluten-Free Beverages

Taste the Dream

www.bloodsugarsolution.com/tastethedream

Soy and rice milk and ice creams.

WhiteWave

www.bloodsugarsolution.com/silksoymilk

Silk soy milk beverage.

WholeSoy & Co.

www.bloodsugarsolution.com/wholesoyco

Unsweetened soy yogurt.

Organic Herbal Teas

Choice Organic Teas

www.bloodsugarsolution.com/choiceorganicteas

Organic fair-trade teas.

Mighty Leaf Tea

www.bloodsugarsolution.com/mightyleaf

Artisan-crafted loose teas in biodegradable pouches.

Numi Tea

www.bloodsugarsolution.com/numitea

Numi inspires well-being of mind, body, and spirit through the simple art of tea.

Yogi Tea

www.bloodsugarsolution.com/yogitea

Medicinal herbal teas.

Water

The best water filters are reverse osmosis filters. While they can be more expensive, the investment is worth it as they remove more toxins from your water supply. If your budget won't allow reverse osmosis filters, Brita is a good alternative.

Reverse-Osmosis Filters

www.bloodsugarsolution.com/h2odistributors

Brita

www.bloodsugarsolution.com/brita

THE 10-DAY DETOX DIET TOOLS AND RESOURCES PAGE

For additional information on resources listed in this book, please see below or visit www.10daydetox.com/tools for additional online resources, including:

Health and Testing Resources

- Basic lab tests (lists which lab tests you need to check for diabesity)
- Online versions of *The Blood Sugar Solution* Diabesity Quiz, Toxicity Quiz, and Food Addiction Quiz
- The *How to Work with Your Doctor to Get What You Need* downloadable guide
- Testing tools (including BMI calculator, glucose monitors, FitBit Wi-Fi Smart Scale, blood pressure monitors, and personal movement trackers)
- The 10-Day Detox Online Health Tracker and Online Journal
- The 10-Day Detox Supplements
- The 10-Day Detox Diet Coaching App
- The 10-Day Detox Diet Tool Kit for Success

10-Day Detox Community Resources

- The 10-Day Detox Challenge
- The 10-Day Detox Community
- How to find a local food co-op
- Life coaching resources

Lifestyle Resources

- Exercise and yoga resources
- The *UltraCalm* guided relaxation program

- Meditation and breathing resources
- Herbal resources
- Stress Management Guide

Food and Nutrition Guides, Support, and Meals

- Access to nutrition coaching support
- Downloadable 10-Day Detox Diet Shopping List
- Brand recommendations for Emergency Life Pack
- The *Restaurant Rescue Guide*
- The 10-Day Detox Diet Vegetarian and Vegan Guide
- Luvo's 10-Day Detox Meals (delicious frozen home meals): luvoinc
  .com/10-day-detox

General Index

ACCU-CHEK Aviva Blood Glucose
    Meter with Strips, 19
additives, 33, 34
alcohol, 34, 39
almond flour, 46
Alzheimer's disease, 28
amino acids, 38
antibiotics, 34, 44
arrowroot, 46
aspartame, 33
autoimmune diseases, 12
autolyzed yeast extract, 32

beans, avoiding, 39
belly fat, 4, 9, 10, 12, 29, 33
blood pressure
    blood pressure cuffs, 18, 19
    high blood pressure, 3, 9, 11, 12, 18, 23
blood pressure cuffs, 18, 19
blood sugar
    balancing, 9, 17, 29, 35, 40, 56
    fiber and, 35–36
    high levels of, 10, 11, 12, 23, 28–29
    medications for, 18
    tests for, 19–20
The Blood Sugar Solution 10-Day Detox Diet
    (Hyman), 3–4, 7, 17
Blood Sugar Solution 10-Day Detox Diet
    Frozen Meals, 30
BMI (Body Mass Index)
    tracking results and, 18–19
    weight and, 12, 18
brain chemistry, 3, 4, 17
breads, 28–29, 32

broiling, meats and seafood, 59
Brownell, Kelly, 10
budgeting, 55–56

caffeine, 34, 39–40
calories, 10, 28, 39, 57
cancer, 4
canned foods, 54
carbohydrates
    cravings for, 4, 12
    fast-acting carbohydrates, 28–29
    on food labels, 34, 35–36
    refined carbohydrates, 3, 4, 10, 12
    slow-acting carbohydrates, 29, 36
Cascadian Farm, 54
casein, 34
chia seeds, 46
chicory root fiber, 36
cholesterol
    diabesity and, 11, 20
    on food labels, 36–37
    HDL cholesterol, 12, 20, 35
    insulin levels and, 4
    LDL cholesterol, 20, 35
    levels of, 4, 11, 23
    NMR lipid (cholesterol) profile, 20
chronic disease, 4, 12–15, 23, 40
"Clean Fifteen" list, 42
coconut aminos, 46
coconut butter, 46
coconut cream, 47
coconut flour, 47
coconut milk, 47
coconut oil, 47

colorings, 33
community-supported agriculture (CSA),
    42, 56
condiments, ingredients of, 33
conversations, mealtime, 25–28
cooking. *See also* kitchen
    budgeting, 55–56
    dinner conversations and, 25–28
    family kitchen and, 24–25
    kitchen tool essentials, 52–53
    meats and seafood, 59–60
    nutrition and, 28–29
    pantry staples, 44–50
    planning meals, 54–55
    reasons for, 22–24
    shortcuts and time savers, 53–54
    using recipes and, 61–62
    vegetables, 58–59
corn, as grain, 46
Costco, 56
cravings
    diabesity and, 12
    elimination of, 4, 17, 28, 29, 60
    food addiction and, 9, 10, 11
    gluten and, 34
    glycemic index and, 29
    proteins preventing, 35

dairy products
    avoiding, 39
    on food labels, 34
dementia, 4
depression, 12
diabesity
    cholesterol and, 11, 20
    definition of, 10
    processed food and, 37
    quiz on, 11–12
    risk factors for, 19
diabetes
    gestational diabetes, 12
    pre-diabetes, 10, 11, 12, 19, 23
    prevalence of, 23
    reversing, 3, 9
    Standard American Diet and, 3
    type 2 diabetes, 4, 10, 11, 12, 20, 28, 40
digestion, 9, 12, 33, 36, 39
dinner conversations, 25–28
"Dirty Dozen" list, 41–42

eggs
    resources for, 314–15
    selection of, 43–44
emotions, 9, 11
energy, 9, 17
energy bars, 32
environmental toxins, 40, 41
Environmental Working Group (EWG),
    22, 40, 41, 44, 56
essential amino acids, 38
essential fatty acids, 48
ethnic groups, 11, 19
exercise, 12

Facebook, 24
farmers' markets, 42, 56
fatigue, 12
fats
    bad fats, 33
    on food labels, 35
    healthy fats, 29, 30
    high-quality fats, 28
    hydrogenated fats, 33, 39, 49
    omega-3 fats, 34, 35, 44, 48
    omega-6 fats, 34
    in packaged food, 23, 33
    snacks and, 57
    trans fat, 33, 35
fertilizers, 34, 41
fiber
    on food labels, 34, 35–36
    levels of, 30
fish. *See also* seafood
    resources on, 315
flaxseed meal, 47
FLC (feel like crap) syndrome, 9, 12
flour
    almond flour, 46
    coconut flour, 47
    food addiction and, 9
    nutrition and, 28–29
food. *See also* nutrition; organic foods;
        packaged foods; processed food; snack
        foods
    as medicine, 4, 7, 17, 40
food addiction
    cravings and, 9, 10, 11
    FLC (feel like crap) syndrome and, 9
    quiz on, 10–11

release of, 17
   sugar and, 7, 9
Food and Drug Administration (FDA),
   33, 39
food industry, 3, 11, 22, 23–24,
   31, 33
food labels
   ingredients list, 32–34, 36
   "Nutrition Facts" section, 34–38
   reading, 31, 32–38, 54
foodlike substances, 38
fried foods, 39
frozen fruits, 42, 55
frozen meals, 23, 30
frozen vegetables, 42, 54, 55
fruits
   as carbohydrates, 29
   "Clean Fifteen" list, 42
   "Dirty Dozen" list, 41–42
   frozen fruits, 42, 55
   low-glycemic index, 42–43
   selection of, 41–43

gas, sweeteners causing, 33
gestational diabetes, 12
glucose monitors, 18, 19
gluten
   avoiding, 39
   on food labels, 34
   nondairy, gluten-free beverages, 317
glycemic index (GI)
   fruits and vegetables and, 42–43
   snack foods and, 28–29
"Good Food on a Tight Budget"
   (Environmental Working Group), 56
grains, avoiding, 39, 46
grapeseed oil, 48
grass-fed meats, 43
grilling, meats and seafood, 59
gut bacteria, 33, 39

Handel Group, 25
Handel Method, 25
HDL cholesterol, 12, 20, 35
headaches, 9, 12
healthcare providers, 18, 20
health claims, 32
heart disease, 12, 28
height, tracking results, 18

Hemoglobin A1c test, 20
hemp protein powder, 48
hemp seed, 48
herbs, 29, 30
high blood pressure, 3, 9, 11, 12,
   18, 23
high-fructose corn syrup, 32, 33
hormones
   balancing, 9, 17
   environmental toxins and, 40
   insulin as fat storage hormone, 4
   in meats, 44
   processed food and, 23
hunger
   caffeine and, 40
   food addiction and, 9, 10
   glycemic index and, 29
   nutritional content of food and, 28
   snacks and, 56
   visceral adipose tissue and, 3, 4
hydrogenated fats, 33, 39, 49

Immuno Laboratories, 12
Immuno Symptom Checklist, 12
impulse control, 39
industrial chemicals, 40
industrial food system, 3, 11, 22, 23–24,
   31, 33
infertility, 12
inflammation, 9, 11, 28, 29, 34, 39, 41
ingredients list
   on food labels, 32
   ingredients to avoid, 32–34
   marketing and, 36
Instagram, 24
insulin
   as fat storage hormone, 4
   high levels of, 4, 9, 28, 33, 37
   insulin resistance, 12
   insulin response test, 20
   triggers for, 10
inulin, 36

Japanese people, sodium consumption
   of, 37
jarred foods, 54
joint pain, 12
journal, for tracking results, 17, 18, 21
junk foods, 38

kelp noodles, 48
kitchen
    family kitchen, 24–25
    items permanently eliminated
        from, 39
    items to avoid, 39–40
    kitchen tool essentials, 52–53
    meats and proteins for, 43–44
    pantry staples, 44–50
    produce for, 41–43
    replacement chart, 50–51
    as safe zone, 31
    stocking with fresh food, 40–51, 44
konjac root, 50

LabCorp, 20
label reading, guidelines for, 31,
    32–38, 54
LDL cholesterol, 20, 35
leaky gut, 39
leftovers, 53
LipoScience, 20
liver, 17
local produce, 42
Ludwig, David, 3
Luvo, 23, 30, 61

maltodextrin, 32
margarine, 39
marketing
    food labels and, 36
    health claims and, 32
mayonnaise, 48
meals
    brunch ideas, 306
    frozen meals, 23, 30
    lunch and dinner ideas, 305–6
    planning meals, 54–55
mealtime, dinner conversations, 25–28
measurements, tracking results with,
    18–19
"Meat Eater's Guide" (Environmental
    Working Group), 44
meats
    broiling or grilling, 59
    resources on, 314–15
    sautéing, 60
    selection of, 43–44
medications, 18

metabolism
    boosting, 9, 17, 28, 29, 39
    resetting, 7
    slowing down of, 4, 10, 33
migraines, 9
minerals, on food labels, 38
miso, 44, 49
Mitchell, John, 61
monitoring devices, 18
monk fruit, 33
monounsaturated fats, 35
mood, 9, 11
MSG (monosodium glutamate), 33
muscle, proteins building, 35
mustard, 49

National Resources Defense Council, 44
natural flavorings, 33
NMR lipid (cholesterol) profile, 20
nonessential amino acids, 38
nonstarchy vegetables, 28, 29, 42–43, 57
nonwhite ancestry, 11, 19
noodles
    kelp noodles, 48
    shirataki noodles, 50
NutraSweet, 33
nutrition
    cooking and, 28–29
    diversity as key to, 38
"Nutrition Facts," on food labels,
    34–38
nuts. *See also* seeds
    as carbohydrates, 29
    resources on, 315–16
    as snack, 28

obesity, 3, 4, 19, 22, 23, 40
obesogens, 40
oils
    coconut oil, 47
    grapeseed oil, 48
    refined cooking oils, 39
    resources on, 315–16
oligofructose, 36
omega-3 fats, 34, 35, 44, 48
omega-6 fats, 34
organic foods
    "Dirty Dozen" list and, 41–42
    meats and proteins and, 43–44

preference for, 42
resources on, 313–14

packaged foods
    added fibers in, 36
    reading food labels, 31, 32–38, 54
    rules for purchasing, 31–32
    sodium in, 37
    toxic food environment and, 23
    trans fat in, 33
palm shortening, 49
pancreas, 17
PCOS (polycystic ovarian syndrome), 12
pesticides, 34, 40, 41
phytochemicals, 40
phytonutrients, 29, 30, 49
polycystic ovarian syndrome
    (PCOS), 12
polydextrose, 36
polyunsaturated fats, 35
potassium, 37
poultry
    cooking, 59–60
    resources on, 314–15
    selection of, 43–44
pre-diabetes, 10, 11, 12, 19, 23
prepared foods, avoiding, 39
preservatives, 33, 34
processed food
    cost of, 55
    elimination of, 31
    food addiction and, 9
    food labels and, 33, 34, 37
    hormones and, 23
    soy in, 38
produce
    resources on, 313
    selection of, 41–43
proteins
    food labels and, 34–35, 37–38
    nutrition and, 28, 29
    resources on, 314–15
    selection of, 43–44
    snacks and, 57

quizzes
    diabesity quiz, 11–12
    food addiction quiz, 10–11
    Toxicity Quiz, 12–15

refined carbohydrates, 3, 4, 10, 12
refined cooking oils, 39
resistant starch, 36
resources
    fish, 315
    frozen and canned foods, 314
    general resources, 312–18
    from Mark Hyman, 311–12
    meats, poultry, and eggs, 314–15
    nondairy, gluten-free beverages, 317
    nuts, seeds, and oils, 315–16
    organic foods, 313–14
    organic herbal teas, 317
    spices, seasonings, sauces, soups, 316
    Thrive Market, 5, 44
    on 10-Day Detox Diet, 318–19
    water, 317–18
rheumatoid arthritis, 9
Rudd Center for Food Policy and Obesity,
    Yale University, 10

SAD (Standard American Diet), 3
salt, 23, 37, 49
saturated fats, 35
sautéing
    meats and seafood, 60
    vegetables, 58–59
SaveOnLabs, 20
sawdust, 36
seafood
    cooking, 59–60
    resources on, 315
    selection of, 44
sea salt, 49
seasonal produce, 42
seasonings, 29, 30, 37
seaweed, 50
seeds. *See also* nuts
    as carbohydrates, 29
    chia seeds, 46
    resources on, 315–16
serving size, on food labels, 35
sex drive, 12
sexual dysfunction, 12
shirataki noodles, 50
shopping lists, 55
shortening, 39
Sidwell, Steve, 61
sleep, 9

snack foods
    glycemic index of, 28–29
    healthy snacking, 56–57
sodium. *See also* salt
    on food labels, 37
sodium-to-potassium ratio, 37
sorbitol, 33
soy
    in processed foods, 38
    selection of, 44
soy protein isolates, 38
spices, 29, 30, 56, 316
Splenda, 33
sports beverages, 32
Standard American Diet (SAD), 3
steaming vegetables, 58
stevia, 33
sucralose, 33
sugar
    avoiding, 32–33
    calories from, 10
    cravings for, 4, 12
    food addiction and, 7, 9
    food labels and, 34
    toxic food environment and, 23
    visceral adipose tissue and, 3
sugar alcohols, 33
supermarket
    layout of, 23
    voting with your wallet, 23–24
Sustainable Seafood Guide (National
    Resources Defense Council), 44
sweeteners, 33
symptoms, Toxicity Quiz, 12–15

tamari, 50
television, 24
tempeh, 44
10-Day Detox Diet
    foods to avoid, 38–40
    getting started, 16–21
    ingredients to avoid, 32–33
    introduction to, 3–4
    length of, 17
    Prep Phase, 16, 31
    principles of, 4–5, 56
    purpose of, 9–15
    resources on, 318–19
    as right-carb diet, 29

10-Day Detox Phase, 16, 39–40
    tracking results, 17–19
    Transition Phase, 5, 16, 31, 39, 54,
      306–7
tests
    blood sugar tests, 19–20
    lab tests, 20
Thai fish sauce, 50
thermogenesis, 39
Thrive Market, 5, 44
tofu, 38, 44
Toxicity Quiz, 12–15
trace ingredients, 32, 33
tracking results
    baseline measurements, 18–19
    blood sugar tests, 19–20
    journal for, 17, 18, 21
    lab tests, 20
    online tools for, 21
Trader Joe's, 56
trans fat, 33, 35
triglycerides, 11, 12, 20
type 2 diabetes, 4, 10, 11, 12, 20,
    28, 40

umami, 49
U.S. Department of Agriculture
    (USDA), 44

VAT (visceral adipose tissue), 3–4
vegetables
    "Clean Fifteen" list, 42
    "Dirty Dozen" list, 41–42
    frozen vegetables, 42, 54, 55
    low-glycemic index, 42–43
    nonstarchy vegetables, 28, 29,
      42–43, 57
    sautéing, 58–59
    selection of, 41–43
    steaming, 58
veggie burgers, 38
visceral adipose tissue (VAT), 3–4
vitamins, on food labels, 38
vitamin water, 38

waist size, tracking results, 18
water
    resources on, 317–18
    vitamin water, 38

weight
    BMI and, 12, 18
    factors increasing weight gain, 22, 34, 39, 40, 53
    factors reversing weight gain, 28
    food as medicine and, 17
    losing weight, 3, 9, 17, 20, 28, 50, 55
    obesity and, 3, 4, 19, 22, 23, 40
    overweight, 12, 18, 23
    tracking results and, 18–19
    trouble losing weight, 4, 9, 12, 16, 40
wheat dextrin, 36

xanthan gum, 32
xylitol, 33

Zander, Lauren, 25, 28

Recipe Index

Açai Smoothie, 66
aioli, Steamed Vegetables with Lemon
    Aioli, 267
almonds
    Almond–Berry Smoothie, 68
    Almond Chicken Salad, 105
    Broiled Salmon with Almond-Dill
        Sauce, 151–52
    Chicken Spring Rolls with Almond
        Sauce, 121–22
    Cocoa-Almond Smoothie, 69
    Coconut Curry Chicken Soup with
        Almonds, 206–7
    Green Beans and Almonds, 254
    Gremolata with Almonds, 292
    Poached Chicken with Coleslaw,
        Almonds, and Pepitas, 186–87
    Strawberry-Almond-Coconut Smoothie, 64
artichokes
    Poached Eggs over Spinach with Braised
        Artichoke Bottoms, 80–81
    Roasted Vegetables with Artichoke
        Hummus, 278–79
arugula
    Arugula and Fennel Salad, 252
    Chipotle Salmon with Arugula Salad,
        160–61
Asian-Spiced Salmon Cakes, 163–64
Asian-Style Beef Stew, 221
asparagus
    Asparagus and Mushroom Frittata with
        Tomato Coulis, 75–76
    Blanched Asparagus with Soft-Boiled
        Eggs, 88

Crustless Asparagus Quiche, 70
    Roasted Salmon and Asparagus with
        Herb-Avocado Mash, 156–57
    Spinach-Mushroom-Asparagus Strata,
        82–83
avocado
    Gua-Kale-Mole, 285
    Roasted Salmon and Asparagus with
        Herb-Avocado Mash, 156–57
    Salmon Burgers with Pickled Radishes and
        Avocado, 154–55
    Spicy Tomatillo-Avocado Sauce, 296
    Thai Tofu and Avocado Salad with
        Chile-Lime Dressing, 90

Baba Ghanoush, 283
Baked Meatballs with Cauliflower Puree,
    222–23
Balsamic Chicken with Sautéed Brussels
    Sprouts, 177–78
basil
    Grilled Chicken with Basil Pesto, 181–82
    Miso-Marinated Cod with Fresh Basil and
        Bok Choy, 170
    Tomato-Basil Soup with Shrimp,
        128–29
beef
    Asian-Style Beef Stew, 221
    Baked Meatballs with Cauliflower Puree,
        222–23
    Beef Bolognese, 239–40
    Beef Chili, 217–18
    Chipotle-Rubbed Steak Salad with Onions
        and Peppers, 224–25

beef *(cont.)*
 Filet Mignon with Garlic Sauce and
  Roasted Tomatoes, 226–27
 Herb-Crusted Beef Tenderloin, 229–30
 Mexican "Rice" Bowl, 237–38
 Rib-Eye Steaks with Grilled Radicchio,
  228
 Slow-Cooked Brisket with Fennel and
  Onions, 219–20
 Slow-Cooked Short Ribs with Celery
  Root Puree, 231–32
 Spice-Rubbed Beef Filet with Braised
  Green Beans and Mushrooms, 233–34
 Taco Salad with Flank Steak, 124–25
Bell Pepper Mini Quiches, 277
Bison Steaks with Wild Mushroom Sauce
 and Haricots Verts, 235–36
Blanched Asparagus with Soft-Boiled
 Eggs, 88
blueberries, Blueberry-Nut Smoothie, 65
bok choy
 Bok Choy Stir-Fry with Black Cod,
  168–69
 Miso-Marinated Cod with Fresh Basil and
  Bok Choy, 170
Braised Broccoli with Tomatoes and Roasted
 Garlic, 260
Braised Celery Hearts in Walnut Oil, 270
Braised Chicken with Onions and Peppers,
 173–74
breakfast
 Açai Smoothie, 66
 Almond-Berry Smoothie, 68
 Asparagus and Mushroom Frittata with
  Tomato Coulis, 75–76
 Blueberry-Nut Smoothie, 65
 Cocoa-Almond Smoothie, 69
 Creamy Berry Smoothie, 67
 Crustless Asparagus Quiche, 70
 Poached Eggs over Spinach with Braised
  Artichoke Bottoms, 80–81
 Southwestern Vegetable Frittata, 73–74
 Spicy Scrambled Tofu with Zucchini and
  Cilantro, 84
 Spinach-Mushroom-Asparagus Strata,
  82–83
 Strawberry-Almond-Coconut
  Smoothie, 64
 Turkey Sausage Patties, 79

 Vegetable Hash with Fried Eggs, 71–72
 Wild Mushroom and Leek Frittata,
  77–78
broccoli
 Braised Broccoli with Tomatoes and
  Roasted Garlic, 260
 Broccoli Tofu, 131–32
 Brussels Sprouts and Broccoli Slaw with
  Seared Scallops, 91–92
broccolini, Garlic and Chile Broccolini with
 Soft-Boiled Eggs, 261–62
broccoli rabe
 Broccoli Rabe with Hot Italian Sausage,
  263
 Turkey Piccata with Brussels Sprout Leaves
  and Broccoli Rabe, 215–16
Broiled Salmon with Almond-Dill Sauce,
 151–52
Brussels sprouts
 Balsamic Chicken with Sautéed Brussels
  Sprouts, 177–78
 Brussels Sprouts and Broccoli Slaw with
  Seared Scallops, 91–92
 Shredded Brussels Sprouts with Warm
  Walnut Dressing, 255
 Turkey Piccata with Brussels Sprout Leaves
  and Broccoli Rabe, 215–16

cabbage
 Chicken Yakitori with Napa Cabbage
  Slaw, 119–20
 Tandoori Shrimp with Indian-Spiced
  Cabbage, 145–46
Caesar Salad with Grilled Chicken, 106–7
cardamom, Zucchini Ribbons with Pearl
 Onions and Cardamom, 268–69
carrots, Chili-Spiced Turkey Meatloaf with
 Roasted Carrot Salad, 210–11
cashews
 Cashew "Ricotta Cheese", 295
 Lemony Cashew-Tahini Dip, 288
 Roasted Vegetable Lasagna with Cashew
  "Ricotta", 133–34
cauliflower
 Baked Meatballs with Cauliflower Puree,
  222–23
 Cauliflower "Rice", 264
 Mashed Cauliflower with Horseradish, 265
 Spicy Cauliflower Sauté, 259

cayenne, Cinnamon and Cayenne Roasted Mixed Nuts, 286

celery, Pan-Roasted Chicken Thighs with Celery Salad and Mustard Vinaigrette, 109

celery hearts, Braised Celery Hearts in Walnut Oil, 270

celery root, Slow-Cooked Short Ribs with Celery Root Puree, 231–32

Cherry Tomato and Tofu Salad, 89

chicken

    Almond Chicken Salad, 105

    Balsamic Chicken with Sautéed Brussels Sprouts, 177–78

    Braised Chicken with Onions and Peppers, 173–74

    Caesar Salad with Grilled Chicken, 106–7

    Chicken Provençal with Zucchini and Peppers, 189–90

    Chicken Salad in Endive Cups, 108

    Chicken Satay with Cucumber Salad, 114–15

    Chicken Spring Rolls with Almond Sauce, 121–22

    Chicken with Oven-Roasted Tomatoes, 183

    Chicken Yakitori with Napa Cabbage Slaw, 119–20

    Chinese Chicken Salad, 118

    Coconut Curry Chicken Soup with Almonds, 206–7

    Forty-Clove Baked Chicken with Swiss Chard, 179–80

    Ginger-Lemon Chicken with Spinach, 202–3

    Grilled Chicken with Basil Pesto, 181–82

    Moroccan Chicken and Vegetable Stew, 175–76

    Moroccan-Style Chicken, 204–5

    Pan-Roasted Chicken Thighs with Celery Salad and Mustard Vinaigrette, 109

    Pan-Roasted Chicken with Wild Mushroom Ragout, 184–85

    Poached Chicken with Coleslaw, Almonds, and Pepitas, 186–87

    Pomegranate Chicken, 188

    Ratatouille with Roasted Chicken, 191–92

    Red Curry Stew with Chicken and Eggplant, 200–201

    Southwestern Chicken Wraps, 193

    Thai Chicken Noodle Soup, 130

    Thai Chicken Salad, 116–17

    Tomatillo Chicken, 194–95

    Tuscan Chicken Cacciatore, 196–97

    Yellow Curry with Chicken Meatballs, 198–99

chili. *See* soups and stews

Chili-Spiced Turkey Meatloaf with Roasted Carrot Salad, 210–11

Chimichurri, 294

Chinese Chicken Salad, 118

chipotle chiles

    Chipotle-Rubbed Steak Salad with Onions and Peppers, 224–25

    Chipotle Salmon with Arugula Salad, 160–61

chives, Shrimp and Three-Mushroom Sauté with Chives, 147

chocolate, Cocoa-Almond Smoothie, 69

cilantro, Spicy Scrambled Tofu with Zucchini and Cilantro, 84

Cinnamon and Cayenne Roasted Mixed Nuts, 286

Cioppino, 139–40

Cocoa-Almond Smoothie, 69

coconut

    Coconut Curry Chicken Soup with Almonds, 206–7

    Coconut Curry with Tofu, 135–36

    Roast Pork Tenderloin with Coconut Curry Vegetables, 249–51

    Sesame-Coconut Curry Sauce, 291

    Strawberry-Almond-Coconut Smoothie, 64

cod

    Bok Choy Stir-Fry with Black Cod, 168–69

    Cod Cakes with Miso Eggplant, 171–72

    Fennel Salad with Roast Cod Fillets, 93–94

    Miso-Marinated Cod with Fresh Basil and Bok Choy, 170

coleslaw, Poached Chicken with Coleslaw, Almonds, and Pepitas, 186–87

condiments. *See* sauces and condiments

coriander, Hot and Spicy Shrimp with Coriander, 150

crab, Thai Green Curry with Soft-Shell Crabs, 143–44

Creamy Berry Smoothie, 67
Creamy Herbed Tahini Dip, 281
Crustless Asparagus Quiche, 70
cucumbers
    Chicken Satay with Cucumber Salad, 114–15
    Cucumber-Kale Smoothie, 272
    Grilled Salmon with Cucumber Salad, 162
    Heirloom Tomato, Cucumber, and Radish Salad, 253
    Sardine-Cucumber Bites, 280
cumin, Tandoori Lettuce Cups with Cumin Sauce, 112–13
curries
    Coconut Curry Chicken Soup with Almonds, 206–7
    Coconut Curry with Tofu, 135–36
    Red Curry Stew with Chicken and Eggplant, 200–201
    Roast Pork Tenderloin with Coconut Curry Vegetables, 249–51
    Sesame-Coconut Curry Sauce, 291
    Thai Green Curry Paste, 302
    Thai Green Curry with Soft-Shell Crabs, 143–44
    Yellow Curry with Chicken Meatballs, 198–99

Deviled Eggs, 274
dill, Broiled Salmon with Almond-Dill Sauce, 151–52
dinner
    chicken and turkey, 173–216
    meats, 217–51
    seafood, 137–72
    vegetarian and vegan, 131–36
Dr. Hyman's Go-To Spice Rub, 301
Dr. Hyman's Super Salad Bar, 85–87

eggplant
    Baba Ghanoush, 283
    Cod Cakes with Miso Eggplant, 171–72
    Red Curry Stew with Chicken and Eggplant, 200–201
    Spicy Garlic Eggplant with Mint, 266
eggs
    Asparagus and Mushroom Frittata with Tomato Coulis, 75–76
    Blanched Asparagus with Soft-Boiled Eggs, 88

Crustless Asparagus Quiche, 70
    Deviled Eggs, 274
    Egg Salad in Endive Spears, 275
    Garlic and Chile Broccolini with Soft-Boiled Eggs, 261–62
    Poached Eggs over Spinach with Braised Artichoke Bottoms, 80–81
    Southwestern Vegetable Frittata, 73–74
    Spinach-Mushroom-Asparagus Strata, 82–83
    Vegetable Hash with Fried Eggs, 71–72
    Wild Mushroom and Leek Frittata, 77–78
endive
    Chicken Salad in Endive Cups, 108
    Egg Salad in Endive Spears, 275

fats, Dr. Hyman's Super Salad Bar, 85–87
fennel
    Arugula and Fennel Salad, 252
    Fennel and Cherry Tomato Salad with Pork Tenderloin, 123
    Fennel Salad with Roast Cod Fillets, 93–94
    Slow-Cooked Brisket with Fennel and Onions, 219–20
Filet Mignon with Garlic Sauce and Roasted Tomatoes, 226–27
fish. *See* seafood
Forty-Clove Baked Chicken with Swiss Chard, 179–80
Fried "Rice" with Shrimp, 148–49
frittatas
    Asparagus and Mushroom Frittata with Tomato Coulis, 75–76
    Southwestern Vegetable Frittata, 73–74
    Wild Mushroom and Leek Frittata, 77–78
fruit
    Açai Smoothie, 66
    Almond-Berry Smoothie, 68
    Creamy Berry Smoothie, 67
    Mixed Berry Salsa, 289

garlic
    Braised Broccoli with Tomatoes and Roasted Garlic, 260
    Filet Mignon with Garlic Sauce and Roasted Tomatoes, 226–27
    Forty-Clove Baked Chicken with Swiss Chard, 179–80

Garlic and Chile Broccolini with
    Soft-Boiled Eggs, 261–62
Roasted Garlic with Olive Oil and
    Rosemary, 287
Spicy Garlic Eggplant with Mint, 266
ginger
    Ginger-Lemon Chicken with Spinach,
        202–3
    Whole Snapper Stuffed with Scallion and
        Ginger, 165
Greek Salad with Spanish Mackerel, 95
green beans
    Green Beans and Almonds, 254
    Roasted Salmon with Green Beans, 153
    Spice-Rubbed Beef Filet with Braised
        Green Beans and Mushrooms, 233–34
greens
    Cucumber-Kale Smoothie, 272
    Dr. Hyman's Super Salad Bar, 85–87
    Forty-Clove Baked Chicken with Swiss
        Chard, 179–80
    Gua-Kale-Mole, 285
    Lamb and Mustard Green Stir-Fry,
        243–44
    Mustard Greens with Grilled Salmon,
        96–97
    Slow-Cooked Salmon with Asian Greens,
        158–59
    Swiss Chard with Pine Nuts and Scallions,
        256
    Tandoori Lettuce Cups with Cumin Sauce,
        112–13
Gremolata with Almonds, 292
Grilled Chicken with Basil Pesto, 181–82
Grilled Salmon with Cucumber Salad, 162
Gua-Kale-Mole, 285

haricots verts, Bison Steaks with Wild
    Mushroom Sauce and Haricots Verts,
    235–36
Heirloom Tomato, Cucumber, and Radish
    Salad, 253
Herb-Crusted Beef Tenderloin, 229–30
Herb Salt, 303
horseradish, Mashed Cauliflower with
    Horseradish, 265
Hot and Spicy Shrimp with Coriander, 150
hummus, Roasted Vegetables with Artichoke
    Hummus, 278–79

Jicama Fries, 271

kale
    Cucumber-Kale Smoothie, 272
    Gua-Kale-Mole, 285
    Kale Pesto, 293

lamb
    Lamb and Mustard Green Stir-Fry, 243–44
    Lamb Korma, 245–46
    Lebanese-Style Lamb Stew, 247–48
    Summer Pesto "Pasta" with Ground Lamb,
        241–42
lasagna, Roasted Vegetable Lasagna with
    Cashew "Ricotta", 133–34
Lebanese-Style Lamb Stew, 247–48
leeks
    Onion-Leek Soup, 126–27
    Wild Mushroom and Leek Frittata, 77–78
lemons
    Ginger-Lemon Chicken with Spinach,
        202–3
    Lemony Cashew-Tahini Dip, 288
    Steamed Vegetables with Lemon Aioli, 267
limes, Thai Tofu and Avocado Salad with
    Chile-Lime Dressing, 90
lunch
    Almond Chicken Salad, 105
    Blanched Asparagus with Soft-Boiled
        Eggs, 88
    Brussels Sprouts and Broccoli Slaw with
        Seared Scallops, 91–92
    Caesar Salad with Grilled Chicken, 106–7
    Cherry Tomato and Tofu Salad, 89
    Chicken Salad in Endive Cups, 108
    Chicken Satay with Cucumber Salad, 114–15
    Chicken Spring Rolls with Almond Sauce,
        121–22
    Chicken Yakitori with Napa Cabbage
        Slaw, 119–20
    Chinese Chicken Salad, 118
    Dr. Hyman's Super Salad Bar, 85–87
    Fennel and Cherry Tomato Salad with
        Pork Tenderloin, 123
    Fennel Salad with Roast Cod Fillets,
        93–94
    Greek Salad with Spanish Mackerel, 95
    Mustard Greens with Grilled Salmon,
        96–97

lunch *(cont.)*
　Niçoise Salad with Poached Salmon, 100–101
　Onion-Leek Soup, 126–27
　Pan-Roasted Chicken Thighs with Celery Salad and Mustard Vinaigrette, 109
　Salmon Salad Wraps, 102–3
　Seaweed Salad with Poached Shrimp, 104
　Shrimp and Snow Pea Salad, 98–99
　Taco Salad with Flank Steak, 124–25
　Tandoori Lettuce Cups with Cumin Sauce, 112–13
　Thai Chicken Noodle Soup, 130
　Thai Chicken Salad, 116–17
　Thai Tofu and Avocado Salad with Chile-Lime Dressing, 90
　Tomato-Basil Soup with Shrimp, 128–29
　Waldorf Salad with Smoked Paprika, 110–11

mackerel, Greek Salad with Spanish Mackerel, 95
Marinara Sauce, 290
Mashed Cauliflower with Horseradish, 265
Mayonnaise, 299
meats
　Asian-Style Beef Stew, 221
　Baked Meatballs with Cauliflower Puree, 222–23
　Beef Bolognese, 239–40
　Beef Chili, 217–18
　Bison Steaks with Wild Mushroom Sauce and Haricots Verts, 235–36
　Broccoli Rabe with Hot Italian Sausage, 263
　Chipotle-Rubbed Steak Salad with Onions and Peppers, 224–25
　Fennel and Cherry Tomato Salad with Pork Tenderloin, 123
　Filet Mignon with Garlic Sauce and Roasted Tomatoes, 226–27
　Herb-Crusted Beef Tenderloin, 229–30
　Lamb and Mustard Green Stir-Fry, 243–44
　Lamb Korma, 245–46
　Lebanese-Style Lamb Stew, 247–48
　Mexican "Rice" Bowl, 237–38
　Rib-Eye Steaks with Grilled Radicchio, 228
　Roast Pork Tenderloin with Coconut Curry Vegetables, 249–51
　Slow-Cooked Brisket with Fennel and Onions, 219–20

　Slow-Cooked Short Ribs with Celery Root Puree, 231–32
　Spice-Rubbed Beef Filet with Braised Green Beans and Mushrooms, 233–34
　Summer Pesto "Pasta" with Ground Lamb, 241–42
　Taco Salad with Flank Steak, 124–25
Mexican "Rice" Bowl, 237–38
mint, Spicy Garlic Eggplant with Mint, 266
miso
　Cod Cakes with Miso Eggplant, 171–72
　Miso-Marinated Cod with Fresh Basil and Bok Choy, 170
Mixed Berry Salsa, 289
mizuna, Wilted Mizuna with Walnuts, 257
Monkfish Tagine, 141–42
Moroccan Chicken and Vegetable Stew, 175–76
Moroccan-Style Chicken, 204–5
mushrooms
　Asparagus and Mushroom Frittata with Tomato Coulis, 75–76
　Bison Steaks with Wild Mushroom Sauce and Haricots Verts, 235–36
　Pan-Roasted Chicken with Wild Mushroom Ragout, 184–85
　Shrimp and Three-Mushroom Sauté with Chives, 147
　Spice-Rubbed Beef Filet with Braised Green Beans and Mushrooms, 233–34
　Spinach-Mushroom-Asparagus Strata, 82–83
　Wild Mushroom and Leek Frittata, 77–78
　Wild Mushroom Sauté, 258
mustard, Pan-Roasted Chicken Thighs with Celery Salad and Mustard Vinaigrette, 109
mustard greens
　Lamb and Mustard Green Stir-Fry, 243–44
　Mustard Greens with Grilled Salmon, 96–97

Niçoise Salad with Poached Salmon, 100–101
nuts and seeds
　Almond-Berry Smoothie, 68
　Almond Chicken Salad, 105
　Blueberry-Nut Smoothie, 65
　Broiled Salmon with Almond-Dill Sauce, 151–52

Cashew "Ricotta Cheese", 295
Chicken Spring Rolls with Almond Sauce, 121–22
Cinnamon and Cayenne Roasted Mixed Nuts, 286
Cocoa-Almond Smoothie, 69
Coconut Curry Chicken Soup with Almonds, 206–7
Green Beans and Almonds, 254
Gremolata with Almonds, 292
Lemony Cashew-Tahini Dip, 288
Poached Chicken with Coleslaw, Almonds, and Pepitas, 186–87
Roasted Vegetable Lasagna with Cashew "Ricotta", 133–34
Shredded Brussels Sprouts with Warm Walnut Dressing, 255
Spicy Roasted Pepper and Walnut Dip, 282
Strawberry-Almond-Coconut Smoothie, 64
Swiss Chard with Pine Nuts and Scallions, 256
Wilted Mizuna with Walnuts, 257

olive oil, Roasted Garlic with Olive Oil and Rosemary, 287
olives, Warm Herbed Olives, 284
onions
    Braised Chicken with Onions and Peppers, 173–74
    Chipotle-Rubbed Steak Salad with Onions and Peppers, 224–25
    Onion-Leek Soup, 126–27
    Roasted Pepper and Red Onion Relish, 298
    Slow-Cooked Brisket with Fennel and Onions, 219–20
    Zucchini Ribbons with Pearl Onions and Cardamom, 268–69

Pacific Coast Bouillabaisse, 137–38
Pan-Roasted Chicken Thighs with Celery Salad and Mustard Vinaigrette, 109
Pan-Roasted Chicken with Wild Mushroom Ragout, 184–85
paprika, Waldorf Salad with Smoked Paprika, 110–11
pepitas, Poached Chicken with Coleslaw, Almonds, and Pepitas, 186–87
peppers
    Bell Pepper Mini Quiches, 277

Braised Chicken with Onions and Peppers, 173–74
Chicken Provençal with Zucchini and Peppers, 189–90
Chipotle-Rubbed Steak Salad with Onions and Peppers, 224–25
Roasted Pepper and Red Onion Relish, 298
Spicy Roasted Pepper and Walnut Dip, 282
pesto
    Grilled Chicken with Basil Pesto, 181–82
    Kale Pesto, 293
    Summer Pesto "Pasta" with Ground Lamb, 241–42
pine nuts, Swiss Chard with Pine Nuts and Scallions, 256
Poached Chicken with Coleslaw, Almonds, and Pepitas, 186–87
Poached Eggs over Spinach with Braised Artichoke Bottoms, 80–81
Pomegranate Chicken, 188
pork
    Fennel and Cherry Tomato Salad with Pork Tenderloin, 123
    Roast Pork Tenderloin with Coconut Curry Vegetables, 249–51
poultry
    Almond Chicken Salad, 105
    Balsamic Chicken with Sautéed Brussels Sprouts, 177–78
    Braised Chicken with Onions and Peppers, 173–74
    Caesar Salad with Grilled Chicken, 106–7
    Chicken Provençal with Zucchini and Peppers, 189–90
    Chicken Salad in Endive Cups, 108
    Chicken Satay with Cucumber Salad, 114–15
    Chicken with Oven-Roasted Tomatoes, 183
    Chili-Spiced Turkey Meatloaf with Roasted Carrot Salad, 210–11
    Chinese Chicken Salad, 118
    Coconut Curry Chicken Soup with Almonds, 206–7
    Forty-Clove Baked Chicken with Swiss Chard, 179–80
    Ginger-Lemon Chicken with Spinach, 202–3
    Grilled Chicken with Basil Pesto, 181–82
    Moroccan Chicken and Vegetable Stew, 175–76

poultry *(cont.)*

Moroccan-Style Chicken, 204–5

Pan-Roasted Chicken Thighs with Celery Salad and Mustard Vinaigrette, 109

Pan-Roasted Chicken with Wild Mushroom Ragout, 184–85

Poached Chicken with Coleslaw, Almonds, and Pepitas, 186–87

Pomegranate Chicken, 188

Ratatouille with Roasted Chicken, 191–92

Red Curry Stew with Chicken and Eggplant, 200–201

Roasted Turkey with Herb Paste, 212

Southwestern Chicken Wraps, 193

Southwestern Turkey Chili, 208

Spiced Turkey and Zucchini Meatballs, 209

Thai Chicken Noodle Soup, 130

Thai Chicken Salad, 116–17

Tomatillo Chicken, 194–95

Turkey Burgers, 213–14

Turkey Piccata with Brussels Sprout Leaves and Broccoli Rabe, 215–16

Turkey Sausage Patties, 79

Tuscan Chicken Cacciatore, 196–97

Yellow Curry with Chicken Meatballs, 198–99

protein, Dr. Hyman's Super Salad Bar, 85–87

quiche

Bell Pepper Mini Quiches, 277

Crustless Asparagus Quiche, 70

radicchio, Rib-Eye Steaks with Grilled Radicchio, 228

radishes

Heirloom Tomato, Cucumber, and Radish Salad, 253

Salmon Burgers with Pickled Radishes and Avocado, 154–55

Ras el Hanout, 300

Ratatouille with Roasted Chicken, 191–92

Red Curry Stew with Chicken and Eggplant, 200–201

red snapper

Steamed Red Snapper and Vegetables en Papillote, 166–67

Whole Snapper Stuffed with Scallion and Ginger, 165

Rib-Eye Steaks with Grilled Radicchio, 228

rice

Cauliflower "Rice", 264

Fried "Rice" with Shrimp, 148–49

Mexican "Rice" Bowl, 237–38

Roasted Garlic with Olive Oil and Rosemary, 287

Roasted Pepper and Red Onion Relish, 298

Roasted Salmon and Asparagus with Herb-Avocado Mash, 156–57

Roasted Salmon with Green Beans, 153

Roasted Turkey with Herb Paste, 212

Roasted Vegetable Lasagna with Cashew "Ricotta", 133–34

Roasted Vegetables with Artichoke Hummus, 278–79

Roast Pork Tenderloin with Coconut Curry Vegetables, 249–51

rosemary, Roasted Garlic with Olive Oil and Rosemary, 287

rubs. *See* spices and rubs

salad dressings

Dr. Hyman's Super Salad Bar, 85–87

Pan-Roasted Chicken Thighs with Celery Salad and Mustard Vinaigrette, 109

Shredded Brussels Sprouts with Warm Walnut Dressing, 255

Thai Tofu and Avocado Salad with Chile-Lime Dressing, 90

salads

Almond Chicken Salad, 105

Arugula and Fennel Salad, 252

Caesar Salad with Grilled Chicken, 106–7

Cherry Tomato and Tofu Salad, 89

Chicken Salad in Endive Cups, 108

Chicken Satay with Cucumber Salad, 114–15

Chili-Spiced Turkey Meatloaf with Roasted Carrot Salad, 210–11

Chinese Chicken Salad, 118

Chipotle-Rubbed Steak Salad with Onions and Peppers, 224–25

Chipotle Salmon with Arugula Salad, 160–61

Dr. Hyman's Super Salad Bar, 85–87

Egg Salad in Endive Spears, 275

Fennel and Cherry Tomato Salad with Pork Tenderloin, 123

Fennel Salad with Roast Cod Fillets, 93–94

Greek Salad with Spanish Mackerel, 95

Grilled Salmon with Cucumber Salad, 162

Heirloom Tomato, Cucumber, and Radish Salad, 253

Niçoise Salad with Poached Salmon, 100–101

Pan-Roasted Chicken Thighs with Celery Salad and Mustard Vinaigrette, 109

Salmon Salad Wraps, 102–3

Seaweed Salad with Poached Shrimp, 104

Shrimp and Snow Pea Salad, 98–99

Taco Salad with Flank Steak, 124–25

Thai Chicken Salad, 116–17

Thai Tofu and Avocado Salad with Chile-Lime Dressing, 90

Waldorf Salad with Smoked Paprika, 110–11

salmon

Asian-Spiced Salmon Cakes, 163–64

Broiled Salmon with Almond-Dill Sauce, 151–52

Chipotle Salmon with Arugula Salad, 160–61

Grilled Salmon with Cucumber Salad, 162

Mustard Greens with Grilled Salmon, 96–97

Niçoise Salad with Poached Salmon, 100–101

Roasted Salmon and Asparagus with Herb-Avocado Mash, 156–57

Roasted Salmon with Green Beans, 153

Salmon Burgers with Pickled Radishes and Avocado, 154–55

Salmon Salad Wraps, 102–3

Slow-Cooked Salmon with Asian Greens, 158–59

Salsa Roja, 297

salt, Herb Salt, 303

Sardine-Cucumber Bites, 280

sauces and condiments

Bison Steaks with Wild Mushroom Sauce and Haricots Verts, 235–36

Broiled Salmon with Almond-Dill Sauce, 151–52

Cashew "Ricotta Cheese", 295

Chicken Spring Rolls with Almond Sauce, 121–22

Chimichurri, 294

Filet Mignon with Garlic Sauce and Roasted Tomatoes, 226–27

Gremolata with Almonds, 292

Kale Pesto, 293

Marinara Sauce, 290

Mayonnaise, 299

Mixed Berry Salsa, 289

Roasted Pepper and Red Onion Relish, 298

Salsa Roja, 297

Sesame-Coconut Curry Sauce, 291

Spicy Tomatillo-Avocado Sauce, 296

Steamed Vegetables with Lemon Aioli, 267

Tandoori Lettuce Cups with Cumin Sauce, 112–13

sausage

Broccoli Rabe with Hot Italian Sausage, 263

Turkey Sausage Patties, 79

scallions

Swiss Chard with Pine Nuts and Scallions, 256

Whole Snapper Stuffed with Scallion and Ginger, 165

scallops, Brussels Sprouts and Broccoli Slaw with Seared Scallops, 91–92

seafood

Asian-Spiced Salmon Cakes, 163–64

Bok Choy Stir-Fry with Black Cod, 168–69

Broiled Salmon with Almond-Dill Sauce, 151–52

Brussels Sprouts and Broccoli Slaw with Seared Scallops, 91–92

Chipotle Salmon with Arugula Salad, 160–61

Cioppino, 139–40

Cod Cakes with Miso Eggplant, 171–72

Fennel Salad with Roast Cod Fillets, 93–94

Fried "Rice" with Shrimp, 148–49

Greek Salad with Spanish Mackerel, 95

Grilled Salmon with Cucumber Salad, 162

Hot and Spicy Shrimp with Coriander, 150

Miso-Marinated Cod with Fresh Basil and Bok Choy, 170

Monkfish Tagine, 141–42

Mustard Greens with Grilled Salmon, 96–97

Pacific Coast Bouillabaisse, 137–38

Roasted Salmon and Asparagus with Herb-Avocado Mash, 156–57

seafood *(cont.)*
    Roasted Salmon with Green Beans, 153
    Salmon Burgers with Pickled Radishes and
        Avocado, 154–55
    Salmon Salad Wraps, 102–3
    Seaweed Salad with Poached Shrimp, 104
    Shrimp and Snow Pea Salad, 98–99
    Shrimp and Three-Mushroom Sauté with
        Chives, 147
    Slow-Cooked Salmon with Asian Greens,
        158–59
    Steamed Red Snapper and Vegetables en
        Papillote, 166–67
    Tandoori Shrimp with Indian-Spiced
        Cabbage, 145–46
    Thai Green Curry with Soft-Shell Crabs,
        143–44
    Tomato-Basil Soup with Shrimp, 128–29
    Whole Snapper Stuffed with Scallion and
        Ginger, 165
Seaweed Salad with Poached Shrimp, 104
seeds. *See* nuts and seeds
Sesame-Coconut Curry Sauce, 291
Shredded Brussels Sprouts with Warm
    Walnut Dressing, 255
shrimp
    Fried "Rice" with Shrimp, 148–49
    Hot and Spicy Shrimp with Coriander, 150
    Seaweed Salad with Poached Shrimp, 104
    Shrimp and Snow Pea Salad, 98–99
    Shrimp and Three-Mushroom Sauté with
        Chives, 147
    Tandoori Shrimp with Indian-Spiced
        Cabbage, 145–46
    Tomato-Basil Soup with Shrimp, 128–29
side dishes. *See* vegetables and side dishes
slaw
    Brussels Sprouts and Broccoli Slaw with
        Seared Scallops, 91–92
    Chicken Yakitori with Napa Cabbage
        Slaw, 119–20
    Poached Chicken with Coleslaw, Almonds,
        and Pepitas, 186–87
Slow-Cooked Brisket with Fennel and
    Onions, 219–20
Slow-Cooked Salmon with Asian Greens,
    158–59
Slow-Cooked Short Ribs with Celery Root
    Puree, 231–32

smoothies
    Açai Smoothie, 66
    Almond-Berry Smoothie, 68
    Blueberry-Nut Smoothie, 65
    Cocoa-Almond Smoothie, 69
    Creamy Berry Smoothie, 67
    Cucumber-Kale Smoothie, 272
    Spicy Mocktail, 273
    Strawberry-Almond-Coconut Smoothie, 64
snacks
    Baba Ghanoush, 283
    Bell Pepper Mini Quiches, 277
    Cinnamon and Cayenne Roasted Mixed
        Nuts, 286
    Creamy Herbed Tahini Dip, 281
    Cucumber-Kale Smoothie, 272
    Deviled Eggs, 274
    Egg Salad in Endive Spears, 275
    Gua-Kale-Mole, 285
    Lemony Cashew-Tahini Dip, 288
    Roasted Garlic with Olive Oil and
        Rosemary, 287
    Roasted Vegetables with Artichoke
        Hummus, 278–79
    Sardine-Cucumber Bites, 280
    Spicy Mocktail, 273
    Spicy Roasted Pepper and Walnut Dip, 282
    Stuffed Campari Tomatoes, 276
    Warm Herbed Olives, 284
snow peas, Shrimp and Snow Pea Salad,
    98–99
soups and stews
    Asian-Style Beef Stew, 221
    Beef Chili, 217–18
    Cioppino, 139–40
    Coconut Curry Chicken Soup with
        Almonds, 206–7
    Lamb Korma, 245–46
    Lebanese-Style Lamb Stew, 247–48
    Monkfish Tagine, 141–42
    Moroccan Chicken and Vegetable Stew,
        175–76
    Onion-Leek Soup, 126–27
    Pacific Coast Bouillabaisse, 137–38
    Pan-Roasted Chicken with Wild
        Mushroom Ragout, 184–85
    Ratatouille with Roasted Chicken, 191–92
    Southwestern Turkey Chili, 208
    Thai Chicken Noodle Soup, 130

Tomato-Basil Soup with Shrimp, 128–29
Vegetable-Herb Stock, 304
Southwestern Chicken Wraps, 193
Southwestern Vegetable Frittata, 73–74
Spiced Turkey and Zucchini Meatballs, 209
spices and rubs
Dr. Hyman's Go-To Spice Rub, 301
Herb-Crusted Beef Tenderloin, 229–30
Herb Salt, 303
Ras el Hanout, 300
Roasted Turkey with Herb Paste, 212
Spice-Rubbed Beef Filet with Braised
Green Beans and Mushrooms, 233–34
Thai Green Curry Paste, 302
Spicy Cauliflower Sauté, 259
Spicy Garlic Eggplant with Mint, 266
Spicy Mocktail, 273
Spicy Roasted Pepper and Walnut Dip, 282
Spicy Scrambled Tofu with Zucchini and
Cilantro, 84
Spicy Tomatillo-Avocado Sauce, 296
spinach
Ginger-Lemon Chicken with Spinach,
202–3
Poached Eggs over Spinach with Braised
Artichoke Bottoms, 80–81
Spinach-Mushroom-Asparagus Strata, 82–83
Steamed Red Snapper and Vegetables en
Papillote, 166–67
Steamed Vegetables with Lemon Aioli, 267
stews. *See* soups and stews
stock, Vegetable-Herb Stock, 304
strawberries, Strawberry-Almond-Coconut
Smoothie, 64
Stuffed Campari Tomatoes, 276
Summer Pesto "Pasta" with Ground Lamb,
241–42
Swiss chard
Forty-Clove Baked Chicken with Swiss
Chard, 179–80
Swiss Chard with Pine Nuts and Scallions,
256

Taco Salad with Flank Steak, 124–25
tahini
Creamy Herbed Tahini Dip, 281
Lemony Cashew-Tahini Dip, 288
Tandoori Lettuce Cups with Cumin Sauce,
112–13

Tandoori Shrimp with Indian-Spiced
Cabbage, 145–46
Thai Chicken Noodle Soup, 130
Thai Chicken Salad, 116–17
Thai Green Curry Paste, 302
Thai Green Curry with Soft-Shell Crabs,
143–44
Thai Tofu and Avocado Salad with
Chile-Lime Dressing, 90
tofu
Broccoli Tofu, 131–32
Cherry Tomato and Tofu Salad, 89
Coconut Curry with Tofu, 135–36
Spicy Scrambled Tofu with Zucchini and
Cilantro, 84
Thai Tofu and Avocado Salad with
Chile-Lime Dressing, 90
tomatillos
Spicy Tomatillo-Avocado Sauce, 296
Tomatillo Chicken, 194–95
tomatoes
Asparagus and Mushroom Frittata with
Tomato Coulis, 75–76
Braised Broccoli with Tomatoes and
Roasted Garlic, 260
Cherry Tomato and Tofu Salad, 89
Chicken with Oven-Roasted Tomatoes,
183
Fennel and Cherry Tomato Salad with
Pork Tenderloin, 123
Filet Mignon with Garlic Sauce and
Roasted Tomatoes, 226–27
Heirloom Tomato, Cucumber, and Radish
Salad, 253
Marinara Sauce, 290
Stuffed Campari Tomatoes, 276
Tomato-Basil Soup with Shrimp, 128–29
turkey
Chili-Spiced Turkey Meatloaf with
Roasted Carrot Salad, 210–11
Roasted Turkey with Herb Paste, 212
Southwestern Turkey Chili, 208
Spiced Turkey and Zucchini Meatballs,
209
Turkey Burgers, 213–14
Turkey Piccata with Brussels Sprout Leaves
and Broccoli Rabe, 215–16
Turkey Sausage Patties, 79
Tuscan Chicken Cacciatore, 196–97

vegan dinners. *See* vegetarian and vegan
    dinners
vegetables and side dishes
    Arugula and Fennel Salad, 252
    Braised Broccoli with Tomatoes and
        Roasted Garlic, 260
    Braised Celery Hearts in Walnut Oil, 270
    Broccoli Rabe with Hot Italian Sausage, 263
    Cauliflower "Rice", 264
    Dr. Hyman's Super Salad Bar, 85–87
    Garlic and Chile Broccolini with Soft-
        Boiled Eggs, 261–62
    Green Beans and Almonds, 254
    Heirloom Tomato, Cucumber, and Radish
        Salad, 253
    Jicama Fries, 271
    Mashed Cauliflower with Horseradish, 265
    Moroccan Chicken and Vegetable Stew,
        175–76
    Ratatouille with Roasted Chicken, 191–92
    Roasted Vegetable Lasagna with Cashew
        "Ricotta", 133–34
    Roasted Vegetables with Artichoke
        Hummus, 278–79
    Roast Pork Tenderloin with Coconut
        Curry Vegetables, 249–51
    Shredded Brussels Sprouts with Warm
        Walnut Dressing, 255
    Southwestern Vegetable Frittata, 73–74
    Spicy Cauliflower Sauté, 259
    Spicy Garlic Eggplant with Mint, 266
    Steamed Red Snapper and Vegetables en
        Papillote, 166–67
    Steamed Vegetables with Lemon Aioli, 267
    Swiss Chard with Pine Nuts and Scallions,
        256
    Vegetable Hash with Fried Eggs, 71–72
    Vegetable-Herb Stock, 304
    Wild Mushroom Sauté, 258
    Wilted Mizuna with Walnuts, 257
    Zucchini Ribbons with Pearl Onions and
        Cardamom, 268–69

vegetarian and vegan dinners
    Broccoli Tofu, 131–32
    Coconut Curry with Tofu, 135–36
    Roasted Vegetable Lasagna with Cashew
        "Ricotta", 133–34
Waldorf Salad with Smoked Paprika, 110–11
walnut oil, Braised Celery Hearts in Walnut
    Oil, 270
walnuts
    Shredded Brussels Sprouts with Warm
        Walnut Dressing, 255
    Spicy Roasted Pepper and Walnut Dip, 282
    Wilted Mizuna with Walnuts, 257
Warm Herbed Olives, 284
Whole Snapper Stuffed with Scallion and
    Ginger, 165
wild mushrooms
    Bison Steaks with Wild Mushroom Sauce
        and Haricots Verts, 235–36
    Pan-Roasted Chicken with Wild
        Mushroom Ragout, 184–85
    Wild Mushroom and Leek Frittata, 77–78
    Wild Mushroom Sauté, 258
Wilted Mizuna with Walnuts, 257
wraps
    Salmon Salad Wraps, 102–3
    Southwestern Chicken Wraps, 193

Yellow Curry with Chicken Meatballs,
    198–99

zucchini
    Chicken Provençal with Zucchini and
        Peppers, 189–90
    Spiced Turkey and Zucchini Meatballs, 209
    Spicy Scrambled Tofu with Zucchini and
        Cilantro, 84
    Summer Pesto "Pasta" with Ground Lamb,
        241–42
    Zucchini Ribbons with Pearl Onions and
        Cardamom, 268–69

About the Author

MARK HYMAN, MD, has dedicated his career to identifying and addressing the root causes of chronic illness through a groundbreaking whole-systems medicine approach known as Functional Medicine. He is a family physician, an eight-time #1 *New York Times* bestselling author, and an internationally recognized leader in his field. Through his private practice, education efforts, writing, research, advocacy, and public-policy work, he strives to improve access to Functional Medicine and to widen the understanding and practice of it, empowering others to stop managing symptoms and instead treat the underlying causes of illness, thereby also tackling our chronic-disease epidemic.

Dr. Hyman is Chairman of the Institute for Functional Medicine, and was awarded its 2009 Linus Pauling Award for Leadership in Functional Medicine. He is also director of the Cleveland Clinic Center for Functional Medicine. He is on the Board of Directors of the Center for Mind-Body Medicine and a faculty member of its Food As Medicine training program, as well as a member of the Board of Advisors of Mehmet Oz's HealthCorps, which tackles the obesity epidemic by educating the student body in American high schools about nutrition, fitness, and mental resilience. He is a volunteer for Partners in Health, with whom he worked immediately after the earthquake in Haiti and continues to help rebuild the country's health care system there. He was featured on *60 Minutes* for his work there.

Dr. Hyman has testified before the White House Commission on Complementary and Alternative Medicine and has consulted with the

Surgeon General on diabetes prevention. He has testified before the Senate Working Group on Health Care Reform on functional medicine and participated in the White House Forum on Prevention and Wellness in June 2009. Dr. Hyman was nominated by Senator Tom Harkin for the President's Advisory Group on Prevention, Health Promotion, and Integrative and Public Health, a twenty-five-person group to advise the administration and the new National Council on Prevention, Health Promotion, and Public Health. With Drs. Dean Ornish and Michael Roizen, Dr. Hyman crafted and helped to introduce the Take Back Your Health Act of 2009 into the United States Senate, to provide for reimbursement of lifestyle treatment of chronic disease. He is an international speaker and presented at TEDMED, the World Economic Forum and the Clinton Foundation's Health Matters Conference, as well as the Clinton Global Initiative America. He continues to work in Washington on health reform, recently testifying before a congressional hearing on functional medicine, nutrition, and the use of dietary supplements.

Through his work with corporations, church groups, and government entities, such as CIGNA, the Veterans Administration, Google, and Saddleback Church, he is helping to improve health outcomes and reduce medical costs around the world. He initiated and is a key participant in the ongoing development of a faith-based initiative that enrolled over 15,000 people at Saddleback Church in a healthy lifestyle program and research study where the congregation lost 250,000 pounds in the first year. In recognition of his efforts, he was recently awarded the Council on Litigation Management's 2010 Professionalism Award, citing individuals who have demonstrated leadership by example in the highest standard of their profession. He also received the American College of Nutrition 2009 Communication and Media Award for his contribution to promoting better understanding of nutrition science. He has been featured on *The Dr. Oz Show, CBS This Morning, 60 Minutes,* CNN, and MSNBC. He was inducted into the Books for a Better Life Hall of Fame in 2015.

Dr. Hyman is founder and medical director of the UltraWellness Center in Lenox, Massachusetts, where he directs a team of physicians, nutritionists, and nurses who utilize a comprehensive approach to health.

Before starting his practice, he was co–medical director at Canyon Ranch Lenox, one of the world's leading health resorts. While at Canyon Ranch, he coauthored the *New York Times* bestseller *UltraPrevention: The 6-Week Plan That Will Make You Healthy for Life* (Scribner) — winner of the Books for a Better Life Award honoring the best self-improvement books each year. He has since written *UltraMetabolism: The Simple Plan for Automatic Weight Loss, The UltraMetabolism Cookbook, The UltraMind Solution, The UltraSimple Diet, The Blood Sugar Solution, The Blood Sugar Solution Cookbook,* and *The Blood Sugar Solution 10-Day Detox Diet,* as well as co–authored *The Daniel Plan* and *The Daniel Plan Cookbook,* all #1 *New York Times* bestsellers. Dr. Hyman graduated with a B.A. from Cornell University and magna cum laude from the Ottawa University School of Medicine. He completed his residency at the University of San Francisco's program in Family Medicine at the Community Hospital of Santa Rosa. Please join him in helping us all take back our health at www.drhyman.com, follow him on twitter @markhymanmd, and see him on Facebook at facebook.com/drmarkhyman.